R. Michels

Training Tomorrow's Psychiatrist

TRAINING TOMORROW'S PSYCHIATRIST

THE CRISIS IN CURRICULUM

edited by Theodore Lidz and Marshall Edelson

New Haven and London, Yale University Press, 1970

Library of Congress catalog card number: 74-99831
Standard book number: (clothbound) 300-0 1207-1, (paperbound) 300-0 1209-8
Designed by Sally Sullivan, set in IBM Press Roman type, and printed in the United States of America by The Carl Purington Rollins Printing-Office of the Yale University Press.
Distributed in Great Britain, Europe, Asia, and Africa by Yale University Press Ltd., London; in Canada by McGill-Queen's University Press, Montreal; and in Mexico by Centro Interamericano de Libros Académicos, Mexico City.

Contents

List of Contributors

Theodore Lidz, M.D., professor of psychiatry, Yale University.

Marshall Edelson, M.D., Ph.D., associate professor of psychiatry, Yale University.

Donald Oken, M.D., professor of psychiatry and chairman of the department of psychiatry, State University of New York Upstate Medical Center at Syracuse.

Seymour R. Kaplan, M.D., associate professor of psychiatry, Albert Einstein College of Medicine.

Preface

Psychiatry has moved a long way during the past thirty years. Prior to World War II there were only some three thousand psychiatrists in the United States, and only a small proportion of them were well trained according to current standards. Not all medical schools had psychiatric curricula, and only a few had programs of any consequence. There was only a handful of good residency training programs and as late as 1950 few, if any, medical schools had more than one full professor of psychiatry. With the help and guidance provided by the Public Health Service the feeble toddler has matured with amazing rapidity, and today there are more than twenty thousand psychiatrists in the country, and departments of psychiatry form major components of virtually every medical school.

The emergence of psychiatry as a major field in medical education was heralded by the 1951 Ithaca Conference on Psychiatric Education [1]. Although it was one of the most successful conferences on medical education ever held, it was concerned not with the training of psychiatrists but rather with the need for and means of providing all medical students with a psychiatric orientation. The 1952 Ithaca Conference [3] focused on the education of psychiatrists, considering in particular residency and post-residency training. The participants at both conferences recognized the serious difficulties created for postgraduate medical education in all fields because graduates of different medical schools had widely divergent educations in psychiatry in contrast to their education in internal medicine, pediatrics, surgery, obstetrics and gynecology. In response to this conference, the Committee on Medical Education of the American Psychiatric Association drafted an outline furnishing minimal requirements of a curriculum for teaching psychiatry in medical schools which was accepted by all but two chairmen of departments of psychiatry prior to its publication in 1956 [2]. The publication of the curriculum was particularly felicitous for it strengthened the requests of many chairmen for more adequate facilities, faculties, and time in the curriculum, and it served as a guide for new medical schools and for those first developing departments of psychiatry.

I refer to these conferences and the publications that resulted from them primarily to point out that careful scrutiny of the educational situation and the preparation of position papers played a notable role in fostering the development of psychiatry in the United States.

We are now facing a new crisis in psychiatric education. The findings of the Ithaca Conferences and the curriculum formulated by the Committee on Medical Education are no longer germane to the current scene. Changes in the health requirements of the nation as well as changes in the field of psychiatry and in medical education require a review and reorganization of psychiatric education.

Despite the remarkable increase in the number of psychiatrists during the past twenty-five years, or perhaps because of it, the demands for mental health personnel have skyrocketed. In New Haven, for example, where there are probably as many psychiatrists per capita as anywhere in the world, the demands for psychiatric services remain insatiable. The national objective of providing adequate medical care for the entire population involves provision for the treatment and prevention of emotional and mental disorders in a wide variety of settings: in general hospitals, in community mental health centers, in various poverty and inner-city rehabilitation programs, in programs concerned with delinquency, crime, and addictions, and so on. With the burgeoning service demands, there is a concomitant increase in the need for sound research to place the therapeutic and prophylactic efforts on a solid foundation. There is, of course, a need for nonpsychiatric mental health workers, but unless they are adequately trained and properly guided, such workers can threaten the integrity of the field and the growing hopes in the efficacy of psychiatry in coping with mental health problems. Serious questions arise concerning the capacities of psychiatrists or psychologists as currently educated to provide the necessary direction and leadership.

We must recognize too that the field of psychiatry has expanded and altered considerably over the past few decades. We can no longer seek to educate psychiatrists who are simply diagnosticians and psychotherapists and who have some reasonable knowledge about running a hospital unit. Psychopharmacology, milieu therapy, group and family therapy, social and community psychiatry, liaison work with other medical specialties, and child and adolescent psychiatry are now among the fields with which a well-trained psychiatrist requires some familiarity and in which he may decide to specialize.

Changes in medical school education also require scrutiny of the teaching of psychiatry. The shortage of physicians has created pressure to reduce the time required for medical education and to increase the size of medical school classes. The federal and state governments can exert powerful influences for increased enrollments because medical schools require financial assistance from them. Some schools have responded by accepting students after two years of college, and most schools are increasing their enrollments. Both measures can be detrimental to psychiatric education. A student requires maturity to be ready to learn psychiatry; and teaching psychiatry properly, even in medical school, requires work in small groups and individual supervision. It is, however, the fundamental revisions in medical school curricula now being instituted that require careful reconsideration of psychiatric education, for some of the curricula open new potentialities. Medical schools are reworking curricula largely because of the growing realization that the medical sciences and the therapeutic techniques have become so complex that it is no longer feasible to prepare all or even most students as generalists, or to give them the proper foundations for specialty training in any field they select after being graduated from medical school. The emerging curricula make it possible, even if not essential, for students to begin their preparation for specialization during the third year in medical school. They have opened the way, as I shall discuss in the first chapter in this volume, for preparing medical students specifically for careers in psychiatry. It is an opportunity for which psychiatric education must be prepared.

The requirements for specialty training in psychiatry include a year of internship in internal medicine, pediatrics, or a "split" or "rotating" internship in several fields, prior to three years of psychiatric residency experience. Recently, the internal medicine and surgery specialty boards decided to count the year of internship in their specialties as part of their residency requirements, thus moving toward virtual abolition of the internship. Such measures have important implications for psychiatric education. The student who intends to become a psychiatrist may have difficulty in obtaining a good medical internship in a university hospital as the places will be reserved for those who intend to become internists. Indeed such difficulties, already reported, require the student to be less than candid about his ultimate intentions. The questions are raised by these circumstances whether psychiatry should continue, and whether it can continue, to require an internship in another field prior to specialization.

I have noted some of the reasons why it has become essential for psychiatric educators to consider changing the education of psychiatrists and, perhaps, changing it drastically. Although individual schools and residency training programs can alter their programs in accord with their needs, facilities, and orientations, some matters require organized planning among schools. Because of problems of medical licensure and specialty certification, and because each residency program depends on many medical schools for the prior education of its residents, certain changes cannot be made by individual schools but require concerted decision and action.

The sectional meeting of the Northeastern Professors of Psychiatry held in New Haven, Connecticut in April 1969, and sponsored by the National Institute of Mental Health, addressed itself to the topic, "New Ways of Training Psychiatrists and Training Psychiatrists for New Ways." The chapters in this book are revisions of papers selected from among those presented at the meeting, focusing on an overview of issues concerning the whole of psychiatric education and then in turn on the special issues arising in medical school education, the internship, and the psychiatric residency. In the first chapter I maintain that current deficiencies in educating psychiatrists cannot be properly remedied by revisions of residency training but require profound changes in medical school curricula to enable some students to prepare specifically for specialty training in psychiatry. I discuss the new curriculum at Yale and how it may alter residency training, and then project the development of a semiautonomous school of psychiatry firmly based in medicine. I also envisage the potentiality of creating a professional career that can bridge the gap between psychiatry and clinical psychology to the betterment of both disciplines. In the second chapter Dr. Marshall Edelson presents a conception of how behavioral science teaching and clinical experience in psychiatry can be integrated in a medical school curriculum organized along the lines of the new "track system" at Yale. He is not offering a prescription or a solution for the practical problems involved in implementation, but presenting rather a conception of the kind of program in which integration of the behavioral sciences and clinical experience might be possible. In the third chapter Dr. Donald Oken considers the question of abolishing the internship by discussing the mixed psychiatry-medicine internship at the Upstate Medical Center at Syracuse. In the process, he provides convincing arguments for continuing some internship experience in a field other than psychiatry, but also indicates that residents are not handicapped by decreasing the time allocated to work in internal medicine. In the final chapter Dr. Seymour Kaplan considers the difficult problem of teaching community psychiatry during the residency training. It is a new field that is currently a source of concern, trial, and experimentation in various programs throughout the country, and the topic is vital to the future of the community mental health centers that are sprouting abundantly as a result of heavy federal fertilization.

The papers included in this volume do not provide solutions nor do they cover all of the significant problems confronting psychiatric educators. They consider some of the significant issues and raise many questions. In a sense, the meeting at which they were given explored the need for new directions in educating psychiatrists, and indicated the need for a conference at which the issues could be examined more fully and definitively.

Theodore Lidz, M.D.

REFERENCES

1. Lidz, T. 1955. The 1951 Ithaca Conference on psychiatry in medical education. *J. Med. Educ.* 30:689-97.
2. _____ (Chairman) and Committee on Medical Education of the American Psychiatric Association. 1956. An outline for a curriculum for teaching psychiatry in medical schools. *J. Med. Educ.* 31:115-28.
3. Whitehorn, J. C., Braceland, F. J., Lippard, V., and Malamud, W. eds. 1953. *The psychiatrist, his training and development: report of the 1952 Conference on Psychiatric Education.* American Psychiatric Association, Washington, D.C.

1: Toward Schools of Psychiatry

Theodore Lidz, M.D.

I believe that the time has come for us to realize that we shall not be able to provide the quantity and quality of psychiatric care required and maintain psychiatry's position of leadership in the mental health field simply by augmenting and modifying our current educational program.

There is a limit to what can be taught during the residency period and we are, therefore, not likely to get very far through revisions of the residency programs alone. The crux of the problem lies in the inadequate preparation of medical students for residency training in psychiatry. We are in a very different position from internal medicine, pediatrics, and surgery. These fields receive residents who have, by and large, obtained a suitable background in the basic sciences fundamental to them as well as a thorough knowledge of pathology and the major disease entities with which they will be involved. These residents have gained familiarity and experience with the provision of clinical care for their patients during their internship. They enter the residency with a solid core of knowledge and with the need for careful immediate supervision behind them; they are already capable of coping with the majority of clinical problems on their own and often have a sufficient overview and depth of knowledge of their fields to select a subspecialty and become meaningfully engaged in investigative work. In contrast the psychiatric residency is a confused period in which boundaries are blurred between at least three major purposes. A good residency program must teach the basic sciences essential to psychiatry as well as the fundamentals needed for clinical work such as psychopathology, psychodynamic theory, and interviewing techniques. At the same time the resident is still learning basic clinical psychiatry and psychotherapy at the level of the novice. And finally he usually becomes involved with some subspecialties before he has gained a proper grasp of the total field and the intricacies of psychiatric work.

The situation cannot be remedied simply by increasing the

number of pertinent courses in medical school and improving their content. The student who intends to specialize in psychiatry requires far more education in the behavioral and neurobehavioral sciences, but the majority of medical students have a limited interest in these subjects and the crowded curriculum cannot provide sufficient time for them. Currently medical schools properly continue to provide all students with a psychiatric orientation, but despite the increasing allotment of time to psychiatry, the curricula treat psychiatry as a minor specialty and do not seek to prepare students to enter it, neglecting the fact that psychiatry is perhaps the fastest growing specialty field and will soon replace pediatrics as the third largest specialty—surpassed only by internal medicine and general surgery. A major segment of each class, between ten and twenty percent of the students in many schools, will ultimately become psychiatrists, and in some schools a similar percentage of students enter with the specific intent of becoming psychiatrists. The difficulty arises because the foundations of a psychiatric education differ substantially from those of all other fields of medicine.

I believe that the time has come for us to start specifically training students for psychiatry while they are still in medical school by offering them a program very different from what they are currently receiving. This will mean a relative neglect of many subjects that are now considered significant to their medical education. I would further propose that we seriously consider moving toward the establishment of semiautonomous schools of psychiatry when we are adequately prepared to do so. Even though we are not ready for this second move, we must consider its feasibility now, for it will take time to institute and in the contemporary world the future is upon us with surprising rapidity.

I wish to make it clear that I consider a medical school education as currently received to be highly valuable for a psychiatrist and essential for those of us who have been interested in neurology or in psychosomatic medicine. However, the question is not whether certain courses are useful or important for a psychiatrist, but rather, whether they are as important as other subjects and experiences that are not now being provided. Medical schools are beginning to recognize that it is no longer possible to prepare all students to enter any field at the end of their medical school education—a realization particularly pertinent to psychiatry where so many topics essential for the preparation of the psychiatrist are either simply indicated or totally neglected in the current curriculum. The years between twenty-one and twenty-six are critical as far as intensity of study is concerned; during this period most persons will probably study more intensively than at any other time in their lives. When I talk to students in the behavioral sciences, I find that some have a breadth of knowledge of the literature in the behavioral and social sciences by the age of twenty-five that few psychiatrists achieve during their lifetimes. During these years the medical student, who probably studies as hard or harder than any other group of graduate students, is spending his time and energy in learning the intricacies of anatomy, pathology, physiology, and physiological medicine; he has only limited time to study what is uniquely human about the human animal living in a social and cultural setting.

Psychiatry, more than any other field of medicine, has its foundations in both the biological and the behavioral sciences. It requires an understanding of the biological basis of human behavior, a grasp of neurobehavioral mechanisms and an understanding of psychopharmacology; and it needs a behavioral science background to understand the essentially human aspects of human adaptation and maladaptation and to comprehend psychodynamic theory. It would be futile, however, to attempt to provide all medical students with the background necessary for the study of psychiatry. We could not maintain their interest or expect to teach these subjects adequately to so large a number. Thus, after providing all students with a common base that is just as essential for internists and surgeons as for psychiatrists, those who have already selected a career in psychiatry will move into a special program during the last half of their medical school education. The new curricula being instituted at Yale, Pennsylvania, Einstein, and Duke open the potentiality for such specialistic preparation during the four years of medical school.

Before discussing the new "track system" at Yale and how it

can affect the education of psychiatrists, I wish to consider the student. Currently many students who have particular competence and interest in becoming psychiatrists are being filtered out by our educational system. While some are being screened out by medical school admissions policies which require college students to spend considerable time in the physical and biological sciences more are eliminated by an educational system that requires students to rescind for a long time a dominant interest in persons and their ways of living. There are many students who are reluctant to spend a large portion of their undergraduate college years competing for high grades in the biological and physical sciences; to devote four years in medical school to many topics not of primary interest to them (which they regard largely as hurdles they must get over in order to become psychiatrists); and finally to spend an additional year in an internship before they ever get into their field of basic interest. I believe such conditions have greatly impeded the proper development of psychiatry, a field where we have an urgent need for students who have a dominant interest in people and in society, its institutions, and its culture.

Because of the reluctance to devote so many years—which to the young seem the best years of their lives—to the study of topics in which they do not have a primary concern, many students turn to clinical psychology, sociology, and the study of community psychology or urbanology, where they can utilize their talents and idealism before these have been throttled by years of study of impersonal topics and by teachers and classmates who derogate their interests and attitudes.

I dare hope that with suitable modifications in medical education that would move the student much more rapidly to topics of particular interest to him and to involvement with people, we will be able to bridge the gap that currently exists between clinical psychology and psychiatry, attracting students to a new educational program and to a somewhat new career.

I have grave concerns over the increasing role of clinical psychology in the mental health field—not out of some blind loyalty to medical education and psychiatry, but rather because I consider that with rare exceptions the clinical psychologist's preparation is just as unsuited as that of the medical student for a career in mental health work. Further, few departments of psychology form suitable settings for the training of clinical psychologists. The academic psychologist considers the clinical psychologist as something of a maverick and often pushes the graduate student into conducting research of pseudopertinence to the mental health field, emphasizing rigorous measurement to the detriment of relevance. Introductory college courses in psychology, with their emphasis on animal experimentation, probably lose more students for psychiatry and clinical psychology than they recruit. I do not think it is a matter of prejudice to say that, by and large, the clinical psychologist has inadequate foundations in the biological bases of human behavior; that he is hampered by his unfamiliarity with medicine and the behavior of ill persons; that he generally lacks adequate experience in the assumption of clinical responsibility, particularly the responsibility for life and death decisions; and that he is unprepared to use the potent and potentially dangerous medications that are now an essential part of modern psychiatric therapy.

On the other hand, the medical preparation for psychiatry also suffers serious shortcomings. After completing medical school, many psychiatrists remain fixated on a medical model of mental disorders. They tend to emphasize disturbances in biological development or in physiological homeostasis as causes of behavioral maladaptations, and consider their patients in terms of illness rather than of personality disorders. The entire social milieu and cultural heritage of the medical school in which he is submerged for four years is detrimental to the proper development of the psychiatrist because of the orientation of his teachers and the paucity of the behavioral science background offered him; and he is very inadequately prepared for the consideration of interpersonal relationships, group dynamics, and societal and cultural aspects of human development and behavior. When he conducts research, he is apt to build upon the basic biological sciences with which he is familiar, rather than following social science models.

What I am writing here has much in common with Lawrence Kubie's proposals for a doctorate in medical psychology [1, 2,

3]. These proposals had much merit, but times have changed and I am not suggesting now that we train medical psychologists who will be engaged primarily in therapy and research. I would rather see a more distinctive type of specialization in psychiatry that still has its foundations in medicine. We can take into account that medical education as a whole is changing; that we now have enough psychiatrists available to teach large numbers of students; and that today it is no longer feasible to train psychotherapists who are not capable of utilizing various medications when necessary and who are unprepared for new developments in neurophysiological and psychopharmacological research.

I now wish to outline the approach to medical education, and specifically to the education of future psychiatrists, that we have been evolving at Yale over the past five or six years. The Curriculum Committee recognized that virtually no students at Yale enter general practice and that a relatively large proportion became investigators and teachers and that therefore it was no longer feasible to attempt to prepare all students to enter all specialties. It had several objectives in mind: it sought a way of increasing the number of medical school graduates who return to the faculties of the preclinical sciences. It wished to involve students with patients and patient care from the start of medical school and increase their awareness of social problems.

As a member of the original committee and then of various subcommittees, I had a special interest in finding a way for the students who entered Yale in order to become psychiatrists to have a curriculum that was more interesting to them and that would better prepare them for their residencies. I shall not dwell on the many problems that arose in finding a plan that could simultaneously foster development of better basic scientists, more socially oriented physicians and more scientifically trained clinicians. In the plan that evolved, the first year and a half is occupied primarily with the basic sciences and the "bridging courses" that prepare for clinical experience (pathology, psychopathology, physical diagnosis, laboratory diagnosis, history taking, and interviewing). A curriculum that confined the basic sciences to the first year, such as has been accomplished at Duke University, was abandoned in the planning stage because it would have eliminated elective work during the first year and left little time for study. However, with the exception of the preclinical courses taught by the department of psychiatry, which were lengthened slightly, the time allotted to each basic science course was shortened.

The department of psychiatry decided to integrate its own courses in personality development, psychopathology, and interviewing techniques into a single course taught in biweekly two-hour sessions during the first semester, weekly two-hour sessions for half of the second semester, and weekly two-hour sessions in the third semester. In this course the first hour of the two-hour sessions is sometimes utilized for a lecture or for the presentation of children or adults to the entire class, but the course is mainly taught in small groups of ten students with two instructors—a faculty member and a resident—in which person-centered or patient-centered discussions focus on a specific phase of human development or some pathology pertinent to it. Lectures have been largely replaced by specially prepared or selected readings, clinical presentations, and seminar discussions. At first the students learn interviewing techniques by watching the instructors interview subjects in the small group, but as the course progresses students carry out the interviews themselves. Television tapes are used and will be used increasingly as we gain experience. This method of teaching requires a rather lavish expenditure of faculty time, but it has been met by considerable enthusiasm from the students and has fostered interest in the person, his development, and his life problems from the week the student enters medical school. We can heartily recommend the utilization of two instructors to teach a group as it has markedly increased the liveliness of interchange.

In addition, two new courses were inaugurated that have particular pertinence in introducing all students to the social background of patients and the social aspects of treatment. During half a semester during the first year, a course in medical ecology is taught jointly by the department of epidemiology and public health and the department of psychiatry, which provides the student with opportunities to meet and interview people in their homes and in institutions in the community surrounding the medical center. Lectures and group discussions provided an orientation to the topic of human ecology and during the past year students visited elderly citizens in their homes under suitable tutelage. The course is new, and a number of problems remain to be worked out, among which are those of properly integrating the orientations of psychiatrists and members of the department of epidemiology and public health.

The second new course, or perhaps I should say the second new experience offered the student, will take place during the summer between the first and second year of medical school. The student will spend six weeks of the twelve-week "vacation" period involved in some type of clinical experience. The types of experience can be quite diverse and have not been fully defined as yet. Students may, for example, work in mental hospitals or psychiatric services, in community health projects, in an Indian Service Hospital, on a hospital unit of any type, in nursery schools, and so forth. The emphasis will be upon experience rather than on some form of direct teaching. However, as the student will have had some preparation for clinical work, we shall experiment with the feasibility of having some students take their clinical clerkships in psychiatry during the summer between the first and second years.

By the end of the fifth semester the students will have completed all of their required clinical clerkships in internal medicine, surgery, pediatrics, obstetrics and gynecology, and psychiatry, and the last eighteen months of medical school will be open for carefully planned elective work. This will consist of a combination of clinical work and further intensive work in the basic sciences. The student will not be free to select random elective courses, but will be expected to spend a substantial part of his time in a program planned by a department or by members of several related disciplines. Some students who are pursuing the goal of becoming members of a preclinical department may spend a larger proportion of their time working in the basic sciences—for example, in biochemistry and cellular biology—whereas others intending to enter a medical specialty will spend more time in some type of clinical work. We envisage students pursuing a major interest and a minor interest—as for example, a student who intends to become a pediatrician may spend most of his time in some type of track prepared by the department of pediatrics and a minor part of his time in the Child Study Center or in psychiatry. While it will be possible for some students to construct programs entirely tailored to their specific needs, it is my personal opinion that a large segment of most students' time will be spent in elective tracks prepared by the various departments or interdepartmental committees. A student may, for example, follow a "track" in the neural sciences, including neuroanatomy, neurophysiology, neurobehavioral sciences, and neurology; or he may focus on an area such as transplants by studying immunochemistry, immunology, and pharmacology while gaining clinical experience in surgery.

In order to maintain the student's interest and further his experience in fields other than those of his selection or specialization, all students will spend approximately a half day each week for one year in general outpatient clinics.

The new curriculum retains the traditional Yale requirement that each student complete a piece of investigative work and write a thesis under the supervision of a faculty member before he can receive his degree. He will now be expected to do his thesis work in a topic related to the track he is following.

Let us now consider briefly what we intend to do in psychiatry during the last three semesters. We are developing a curriculum which will integrate course work in the behavioral sciences, including the neurobehavioral sciences and work in psychopharmacology, with an assortment of intensively supervised clinical experiences, as in the plan presented by Dr. Edelson in the next chapter. At the same time we hope to provide some sort of personal therapeutic experience, presumably group therapy, for those students who are majoring in the psychiatry track.

The track must be so planned that some students, particularly those who intend to enter fields other than psychiatry, can participate in some portions of the track or take some courses without making the psychiatric track their major involvement. The track will provide a concentrated experience for students seeking a solid foundation in fields we consider basic to psychiatry, while also providing considerable clinical experience in a psychiatric hospital, in a general hospital, and in community mental health work. In addition, the student will conduct his own research project under a tutor or supervisor. In the process we hope to train some students who will later make a career out of working in and teaching various behavioral science subjects in a manner suited to psychiatric or medical school education.

I wish to emphasize a major advantage of this plan: we shall no longer be trying to teach all medical students during the last year and a half of medical school but only those who have a dominant interest in what we are seeking to teach. Further, as the program develops we anticipate that students with a particular interest in becoming psychiatrists will enter Yale Medical School in order to participate in the program, which in itself will bring us students more suited to the specific curriculum.

On the completion of this program, the student will have a reasonable familiarity with 1) psychodynamic and psychoanalytic theory and personality development; 2) the neurobehavioral sciences and psychopharmacology, both at a theoretic and practical level; 3) various psychologies of potential pertinence to the field, such as the work of Piaget, operant conditioning, learning theory, dissonance theory, and psycholinguistics; 4) the foundations of sociology, social psychology, and ethnology; 5) techniques and attitudes required for interviewing patients; 6) the various psychiatric syndromes; 7) various types of therapy that will enable him to function as a resident from the start of his residency training.

A curriculum such as this should eventually provide us with a very different resident from the one we have at present and enable us to conduct a very different type of residency—one in which the resident will be more useful in working with patients and will receive better supervision. A larger number of residents will be able to pursue investigative work because less of their time and energy will go into mastering fundamentals and working through the marked confusions concerning orientation that currently obfuscate the residency training program.

Our graduates will be physicians: they will have had clerkships in the major fields of medicine even though perhaps not as extensively as at present in some fields, and they will be able to pass their state licensure boards and at least the first two parts of the National Board Examinations.

The second stage that I envisage in changing the education of psychiatrists is a simple matter, namely, abolishing the requirement for an internship in a field or fields other than psychiatry and replacing it with a psychiatric internship. This change is already in progress at some centers where a split internship is being offered in medicine and psychiatry, which in a few places seems to be turning primarily into a psychiatric internship. A number of medical students who intend to become psychiatrists with whom I have spoken would like to have the opportunity to move into their future specialty more rapidly. Although clinical clerkships have at least partly replaced the need for the internship, which originally had the purpose of augmenting medical school lectures and laboratory experience with a period of carefully supervised work with patients, many psychiatric educators would be reluctant to eliminate a year of intensive work in medicine or pediatrics. The question is whether such work is more important for most psychiatrists than additional concentration on psychiatry. If the psychiatric intern has had concentrated psychiatric clerkship experiences while in medical school, part of his internship can be spent as a psychiatric liaison person on medical or pediatric services. Dr. Oken discusses these problems in his chapter in this volume.

The third stage is still a vision or a dream, but perhaps no longer a dream for a distant future. It can begin to change into a tangible reality if our track system functions well (or if some similar program successfully evolves elsewhere) and when we have gathered the necessary experience in teaching and assembled suitable teachers. The dream concerns the development of semiautonomous schools of psychiatry, specifically oriented to the development of medically trained psychiatrists rather than psychiatrists who are retrained physicians. The program outlined in the current Yale curriculum need not change very greatly. By eliminating the psychiatric clerkship from the first two years of the curriculum and by working six weeks during the summer between the second and third years of medical school, the student will be able to complete all of his clerkships aside from psychiatry. Psychiatric clerkships will then be provided as a part of a more fully integrated program during the last two years of medical school which will then become two years in a school for psychiatrists. I do not yet know what kinds of changes will be made during these last two years, for we require the experience with our track system to enable us to construct a feasible and well-integrated program. However, a major change will take place if only because the student will be fully involved in a school for psychiatrists rather than in a school in which the training of psychiatrists is a subsidiary consideration. He will also be surrounded by students with similar objectives even though they may differ in ultimate specialization within psychiatry.

One objection to this plan is that it requires the student to decide to become a psychiatrist earlier. Currently a number of medical students do not decide upon a psychiatric career until the fourth year in medical school, or even during the internship, and some who enter medical school to become psychiatrists change their minds and enter other specialties. The argument has validity, but it applies to any sort of occupational choice: the law student might have decided to become a clergyman if he had had more experience. In other countries, career decisions are usually made earlier than in the United States, for much depends on the type of secondary school attended; and more specific career decisions are made at the time the student enters the university at the age of nineteen or twenty.

A second objection might be raised that establishing semi-autonomous schools of psychiatry would further separate psychiatrists from their colleagues in other areas of medicine. Of course not all students will enter psychiatry through such schools, at least not at first. However, the basic question concerns whether or not psychiatrists can be educated and trained as well under the present system as in the proposed plan. My own experience suggests that psychiatrists are accepted and sought out by physicians in other fields when they are useful as psychiatrists, when they complement and supplement the other physicians' capacities. I believe that psychiatry differs from the remainder of medicine sufficiently to require a different type of education.

A third concern is that departments of psychiatry would become so involved in educating psychiatrists that the medical student who goes into other fields would be neglected. Although semiautonomous schools would consume much of the time, effort, and attention of the psychiatric faculty, schools of psychiatry would have larger and more diversified faculties than departments now have. Psychiatric residents and junior faculty would be more capable teachers who could assume greater responsibilities in teaching medical students.

Following graduation from the school of psychiatry, the trainee would have a two-year residency. We believe that by the end of these two years of residency training—six years after the individual has completed college—he will be far better trained in general psychiatry than he now is after the completion of three years of residency—eight years after he has completed college. He will then be about twenty-eight years old. This projection takes into account that psychiatry has now become a very broad field and will become even broader in the years to come, and that subspecialization is becoming as imperative as specialization within the general field of medicine. The psychiatrist will then move on to have two years of specialty training in such subjects as child psychiatry, community psychiatry, public health psychiatry, psychopharmacology, and so on.

Training in psychoanalysis presents some special problems. Psychoanalytic education has been under the aegis of psychoanalytic institutes which, with a few exceptions, have not been parts of the university. In general these institutes have sought to educate and train for the practice of psychoanalysis as a specialty. The length of training, the time required each week, and the expense often interferes with academic careers and discourages many psychiatrists from obtaining psychoanalytic education and experience. It may be feasible and useful to provide different types of psychoanalytic education according to whether the student wishes to enter psychoanalytic practice, pursue a different subspecialty, or embark on clinical investigation. The psychiatrist who has been educated in a school of psychiatry will already have considerable knowledge of psychoanalytic theory and the literature. I would hope that after the very special psychiatric education he has received, he would be able to complete his psychoanalytic training approximately three years after finishing his two years of general psychiatric residency. The psychiatrist who intends to become an analyst would, I propose, usually start his personal analysis during his residency, or even earlier. Then, during the three years of specialty training in psychoanalysis, he would have seminars, continuing case conferences, and more intensive supervision of "control" cases than currently. In general, I believe that the candidate's personal analysis should not extend beyond three years. Although it may not have reached a fully satisfactory conclusion, it should permit his training analyst to judge whether or not he can become a competent analyst. He can then resume his personal analysis when it no longer affects his accreditation as an analyst. One of the major problems in psychoanalytic training today is that a proper personal analysis often does not take place because the analysand is being evaluated as a candidate more or less on the basis of the personal analysis.

With the development of schools of psychiatry, psychoanalytic education might finally find its proper home in universities and bring the psychoanalytic institutes out of the isolation that is jeopardizing the future of psychoanalysis by fostering parochialism and emphasis upon tradition rather than scientific curiosity and change. Clearly, many problems are involved in shortening the time required for psychoanalytic training by increasing its intensity, and these cannot be discussed comprehensively here. However, great advantages would ensue if the formal education and supervision were completed when the psychoanalyst were in his early thirties. He could then use his analytic training during his more productive years and would become an independent person at a reasonable age when he is more capable of making original contributions to the field. Properly selected and educated, the psychiatrist need not view the completion of his formal psychoanalytic training as the end of his education.

I wish to note some salient problems in such planning. It is obvious that one medical school cannot move into such marked changes in psychiatric education alone. No residency program wishes to confine its selection of residents to candidates from its own medical school. Then there are problems concerning medical licensure: although the Yale program as currently planned would lead to medical licensure, the establishment of schools of psychiatry might well require licensure of a different type. Then, of course, requirements for board certification in psychiatry would have to be changed to permit the altered educational plan. These are not major stumbling blocks.

Finally, we must consider the significant problems of finding adequate and knowledgeable faculty and sufficient space to carry out such programs. The Yale Medical School and department of psychiatry are relatively well off for faculty capable of conducting such educational processes; but problems such as finding ample space within the facilities of the department of psychiatry for those students specializing in psychiatry have not yet been faced realistically. It is also quite clear that a track program requires a very substantial increase in the time devoted to teaching medical students and requires faculty members who have the majority of their time free for such teaching. The drain will be partially offset by a diminution of the courses required for residents and the greater usefulness of the residents both in caring for patients and in teaching medical students.

These, then, are in broad outline my proposals for bringing the education and training of psychiatrists more in line with current needs and knowledge. The implementation of the general approach suggested would, of course, differ from school to school. These proposals suggest not only a way of increasing the number of psychiatrists but also a means of providing the depth of knowledge and breadth of experience the psychiatrist in his formative years requires. This educational system takes cognizance of the scope of psychiatry as a field and its divergencies from the remainder of medicine. It seeks a way of providing a proper foundation for those who wish to specialize in it.

REFERENCES

1. Kubie, L. S. 1954. The pros and cons of a new profession: a doctorate in medical psychology. *Texas Reports on Biology and Medicine* 12:125-70.
2. ——. 1957. Need for a new subdiscipline in the medical profession. *Arch. Neurol. Psychiat.* 78:282-93.
3. ——. 1964. A school of psychological medicine within the framework of a medical school and university. *J. Med. Educ.* 39:476-80.

2. The Integration of the Behavioral Sciences and Clinical Experience in Teaching Medical Students

Marshall Edelson, M.D., Ph.D.

A NEW CURRICULUM: THE TRACK PROGRAM

At the Yale University School of Medicine, we are—as are so many others—currently preoccupied with the development of a new curriculum. The first two-and-a-half years will include work in the basic sciences and seven clinical clerkships. Following this core curriculum, during the final three semesters in medical school, each student will have the opportunity to choose a special "track" appropriate to his own goals or interests. In choosing, or collaborating in planning, his individual track, the student will be stimulated to try to answer the perhaps impossible-to-answer question, "What will I wish, ten years from now, I had had the chance to learn or delve into more deeply in medical school? What will I find then I need to know that I should study now?" The student's individual track may also grow out of some wish to do intensive work in a particular area no matter what his future plans might be, an intellectual fling, so to speak, before a final commitment—perhaps even to some quite different field. It is not, then, the content of a particular track that will repay the investment in such intensive work, not what facts were learned or what problems studied, but what was learned about the ways in which facts may be regarded or problems approached.

The track will not be designed to train the medical student in some narrowly conceived area of technical competence. The intention is different: a pause before specialization or the hectic practice of a profession; a revisit to the knowledge of basic science, and at the same time an immersion in advanced clinical experience, and the two—rather than existing in isolated compartments, neither one related to, or enriching, the other—coming together within the mind of the medical student.

The goal of the track program is, then, the *integration* of basic science and clinical experience. Such an integration may be manifest in the creation of a physician who is neither a laboratory scientist merely measuring the measurable with precision nor a clinical-service-technician.

The work of such a physician, should he choose to do formal research, is guided by the imaginative questions he seeks to answer. Problems of precision of measurement, rigor of control, and "hardness" of data—rather than being ends in themselves—are subordinated to his quest and solved in terms of that degree of precision, rigor, and "hardness" required by his question and the nature of the empirical system through the study of which it is to be answered [12].

On the other hand, his efforts to develop new skills to cope with complex clinical phenomena are disciplined by an application of knowledge involving rigorous consideration of means-ends relations. Such discipline is also evident in his attempt to control—to whatever extent is possible—the conditions determining whether or not his clinical skills can in fact be exercised. Such disciplined clinical work may in turn give rise to new knowledge, for through such work novel situations are created in which crucial phenomena not otherwise observable are elicited. In my own field, discoveries dependent upon the psychoanalytic situation, or upon group situations involving careful attention to control of system, task, and role boundaries and transactions across such boundaries, come to mind [9, 29, 34].

In the department of psychiatry, we are in the beginning of our planning for a behavioral sciences track. In this chapter, I shall share with you some tentative ideas about the direction such a program might take.

CHARACTERISTICS AND HAZARDS OF THIS HISTORICAL MOMENT

What are the characteristics of the historical moment to which we respond by making such plans? First, the present historical moment is characterized by the increasing rate of generation of new knowledge and introduction of technological innovation. This creates two kinds of strain. One has to do with the continuous demand for reorganization of systems of knowledge to cope with the threat of developing incoherence in such systems. The second has to do with the continuous necessity to reexamine the hierarchy of priorities governing what knowledge is relevant and should be internalized within—and used in processes of action by—action systems (both individual and collective), which, after all, have finite capacities for receiving and processing information.

Second, the present historical moment is characterized by uncertainties concerning the relative value of, and priorities of commitment to, the attainment of various social ends. Related to both characteristics is the breakdown of traditional integrative norms, the blurring and questioning of traditional roles, and the alteration of traditional relationships between individuals and groups.

What are the implications of such processes for curriculum planning? Should we not concentrate on what is most general—methods, principles, system characteristics—rather than on masses of particular, detailed content? Would it not make sense to teach not *what* to think but *how* to think, seeking to convey the unique conceptual and methodological problems that confront the student who is trying to understand particular kinds of phenomena, so that he is eventually able to move around in a field on his own? As a corollary of this, should we not focus on those facts illustrating what is general, or those facts having special significance for theory and, therefore, the discovery of new facts, rather than on a fact for its own sake or even for its specific practical value in here-and-now situations? And as another corollary, should we not emphasize on the skill level the development of attitudes, values, orientations, and skills relevant over a wide range of situations, rather than training in situation-specific techniques? More particularly, in psychiatry, should we not avoid the student's overidentification with particular faculty members, and the competition among faculty for such identification, especially if this will result in an exclusive commitment to *one* empirical system—physiological organism, personality system, or social system—or *one* treatment technique or agency of change, or *one* way of doing research, as solely legitimate for the study and alteration of behavior?

These implications may indeed follow from the frightening, yet perhaps also exhilarating, task confronting us: that we must help bring into being a physician who will be able to function in a world we cannot now conceive, with skills that will be relevant to situations we cannot now imagine, and whose relationships to his patient and to various sectors of society may be governed by what are, in the light of our own norms, unanticipated expectations, contracts, or injunctions.

The hazards of the present historical moment for us lie in our modes of response to the anxieties it arouses. One hazard is constituted by a defensive entrenchment—a refusal to change curriculum or covert attempts to sabotage and resist such change. For example, lecture notes may stay the same despite the endless committee discussions or "firm" decisions about curriculum design or goals. Feelings persist that the medical student must continue to be exposed to certain materials, no matter what difficulties ensue as he tries to absorb an ever growing corpus of additions. The injunction seems to be: add the new, without discrimination; retain the old, also often without discrimination.

Another, somewhat different hazard is constituted by a growing distrust of, and contempt for, knowledge itself. Perhaps one loses confidence in one's own and others' conceptual power to master the increasingly complex and mutable. Such loss of confidence and doubt may become depreciation of knowledge, and of its guardians as well—including oneself as teacher and investigator occupying a role felt to be meaningless for the time in which one lives. As a result, primary responsibility for seeking, maintaining, and transmitting knowledge may be abrogated in favor of actions in other arenas. For example, one may become increasingly preoccupied with demands for service, to the extent that they preempt the resources required for thinking about problems and for creating new patterns of thought and skill as well as maintaining existing ones. One may, still in the guise of one's faculty role, become concerned with power, rather than knowledge, and with determining the ends of society. Or one may commit oneself to moral action aimed at resolving the strains within society, in place of, or sometimes hectically vacillating with, a primary interest in the mobilization and transmission of resources for adaptation. These resources are encoded in the works of man—which are culture—and especially that work of man called science.

These, then, are the hazards we face: we may abandon identity and purpose as teachers and investigators, turning instead to other tasks; or we may, entrenching ourselves in the traditional, merely pass on to our students, with whatever abilities we possess, all our present inadequacies as well.

A PROLOGUE TO CURRICULUM: "SYMBOLISM" AND "SYSTEM"

Every curriculum arises from and maintains a view of man and his works and the principles for organizing knowledge derived from that view. This present attempt to adumbrate the shape of a future curriculum may benefit by a prior consideration of what view of man and his works and what principles for organizing knowledge are implied by our current thinking about a behavioral sciences track curriculum. In turn, the view thus made explicit may guide the further development of such a curriculum. (I realize the following comments will involve us in a digression that may seem pointlessly distracting. May I assure the reader that the digressiveness is only apparent; I believe that it will become clear later in the chapter that this prologue provides us with a valuable frame of reference for considering problems of organizing a behavioral sciences curriculum.)

The key terms in such a prologue to curriculum will be Bertalanffy's felicitous conjunction of *symbolism* and *system:* "We have to define what is specific in human behavior and psychology; this is possible in terms of man's symbolic activities. And against the robot model of the primary reactivity of the organism a new conception emerges which can be termed as that of man as an active personality system" [1, p. 12]. However, before turning to new ways of thinking about man in the behavioral sciences, let us become especially aware of our customary ways of thinking.

These customary ideas are embodied in the doctrines of positivism.

We are witness to the bankruptcy of positivism as a sufficient frame of reference for the behavioral scientist, a bankruptcy made inevitable, paradoxically, by the empirical discoveries of the positivist Freud and, in sociology, by the work of Weber and the positivist Durkheim. This bankruptcy was reported in exhaustive detail by Talcott Parsons in his 1937 work, *The Structure of Social Action,* in which he also outlined an alternative to positivism, the voluntaristic theory of action, and an organization of the behavioral sciences based upon that alternative [25]. Positivism as a frame of reference for understanding human behavior, following Parsons' account, may be defined by the following propositions.

1. The meaning of a proposition is identical with the scientifically knowable totality of external reality to which it refers. In other words, there is an immediate correspondence between reality and the propositions describing it. Therefore, the categories of a particular conceptual frame of reference are adequate to explain all the important facts about any concrete phenomena to which they are applied. An example is the belief that the categories of classical mechanics, or categories derived from these, are completely adequate for the scientific understanding of reality.

2. Action is determined by the conditions of action, that is, by such aspects of the actor's situation as his heredity or his environment. In other words, the causes of action are totally encompassed by the constraints imposed by hereditary endowment and the reactions compelled by environmental stimuli.

3. Consideration of aspects of phenomena within the subjective frame of reference of the actor is contrary to the canons of empirical science. (The subjective aspects of action may also be regarded as mere epiphenomena of the conditions of action.) If action is determined by subjective elements at all, it is determined by valid empirical knowledge or by deviation from such knowledge in the direction of error or ignorance. That is, the actor bases his action on considerations that more extensive knowledge would have shown to be erroneous or he was ignorant of certain

facts and would have acted differently had he known them. Ultimately, positivists believe, the conditions of action (heredity and environment) are responsible for ignorance and error.

4. The ends of action are considered to be random and without significant relation to each other. Interaction is not believed to be governed by a shared system of ends, which are hierarchically ordered according to value priorities. Utilitarian positivism tends, rather, to belief in the adequacy of the mechanism of rational pursuit of self-interest by each to produce the greatest possible satisfaction for all.

In positivism, ends may also be regarded as chosen by the actor –if the verb "to choose" has any meaning in such a frame of reference–according to scientific knowledge of empirical reality (that is, knowledge of the past and present). Action is, therefore, essentially determined by the actor's situation, to which it is a rational adaptation. The "end" of action has no conceptual independence but is assimilated into the conditions of action. This variety of positivism tends to lead to belief in the primacy of the role of reason in human affairs. Men adapt means to achieve ends in the most efficient manner on the basis of knowledge of means-ends relations verifiable by the methods of science. (Therefore, religion, for example, is simply the product of ignorance and error with respect to available scientific knowledge.)

5. In the behavioral sciences, positivism tends to ally itself with a tradition of belief in evolutionary progress proceeding in a linear process to a foreseeable culmination. To the extent that action is considered to be determined by a rational understanding of conditions and guided by the application of knowledge, the result of action will vary according to the state of knowledge. Since there is a progressive accumulation of scientific knowledge, ignorance and error must be progressively eliminated. Social evolution, then, is linear and progressive.

Suppose that, as thorough positivists, we were to eliminate all subjective elements, including rationality, as factors. Heredity and environment become the "causes" of action. Then, if hereditary variations are automatically selected in terms of adaptation to environmental conditions, or if, corresponding to natural selection, there is automatic environmental conditioning of random events according to what is adaptive (rewarding), then social evolution is linear and progressive.

A contrasting and increasingly influential view of man has found one statement in Cassirer's *An Essay on Man* [4]. Man is the *animal symbolicum,* the symbolizing animal. Burke states, similarly, "Man is 'the animal that makes, uses and misuses symbols.' Man is/ (1) The symbol-using animal/ (2) Inventor of the negative/ (3) Separated from his natural condition by instruments of his own making/ (4) And goaded by the spirit of hierarchy" [2, pp. 199-200].

Along the same lines, Parsons has emphasized that men respond not to things as they are but to the meanings things have for them. These meanings may be inferred from men's actions or represented by them in symbols. Men do not merely respond to stimuli but try to fit their actions to patterns deemed by them to be desirable. In other words, men's actions are guided by values and oriented to the actualization of such values through processes of goal-attainment. Men orient themselves and account for the choices they make among available alternatives by reference to motives, feelings, and ideas (nonscientific as well as scientific), which are represented by symbols. Since phenomena have a relevant subjective aspect, a frame of reference within which to describe personality and social systems must be capable of including such subjective aspects of action. In such a frame of reference, normative and expressive elements are crucial in understanding action. These elements interact, however, and are interdependent in specific ways not only with each other but with nonnormative elements, such as the conditions of action, which therefore also have an important role in action. The emergent property of a social system is the existence of a common, more or less integrated, system of symbolized meanings shared by its members. Such symbolized meanings include values and the integrative standards or norms, sought ends, and relevant representations of the object-situation derived from such values [25].

One might here also call attention to Freud's most important discoveries. Despite a positivist belief that psychological phenomena would eventually be completely explained by a neurophysiological conceptual system, a belief he apparently never abandoned, Freud was nevertheless bold enough to abandon a strategy founded on that belief and to study psychological phenomena as if these constituted an empirical realm in their own right for the explanation of which a psychological conceptual system was required. He thereby discovered a realm of symbolic processes, which he called "psychic reality." Psychic reality included symbolic inventions, which neither duplicated external reality nor depended on inputs from external reality for their continued power to generate effects. Of course, representations of actual events were used as materials in the creation of psychic reality, and they might, on particular occasions, activate specific symbolic inventions, giving these increased value as determinants of the interpretation of current experience, the allocation of interest or priority, and the direction of action. Similarly, psychic reality was not a mere effluvium of neurophysiological conditions.

That patients suffer from "reminiscences" was one of Freud's early formulations giving primacy to symbolic process in etiology. This insight was enhanced by his fortunate recovery from his "mistake" in ascribing causal status to supposed actual seductions in childhood: he saw that "mere" phantasies of relationships and events–symbolic processes of a special kind–may also have causal efficacy. Again, in discovering transference, he discovered that concrete social objects in current experience may serve as vehicles for symbolic representation or re-creation of past experience. Both Freud's topographical and structural theories of personality may be regarded in part, at least, as classifications of types of symbolic process and attempts to account for their interaction. The concept "superego" most clearly refers to a symbolic invention, which is not in its origins a simple outcome of "learning from experience" or of constitutional givens, but which coexists as a relatively independent variable together with representations of current experience and the consequences of neurophysiological states. The concept "ego" and "id" seem also to refer ultimately to kinds of symbolic process. The significant theme in Freud's empirical work is a view of man in terms of conflicting motives, as these are manifested in symbolic processes with different characteristics and aims. His discovery and description of two modes of symbolization—primary and secondary process—will probably survive as one of his greatest achievements.

Man's behavior, then, is not merely dependent on his past or present experience. He may, through symbolic processes, create and re-create his past and act partly in terms of his own imagination of it. He is able, through symbolic processes, to imagine future states of affairs and he may expend effort to actualize such an imagined state of affairs. He is able in the presence of "yes" to imagine "no," and in any situation to imagine alternatives and their possible consequences. The imagined world, the world of symbols, is not a simple replication, summation, or extract of experience, but a novel invention which is imposed upon experience.

Man cannot know reality directly; he can know it only through his symbolic representations of it. Such symbolic representations are made with language, but other vehicles and media—including body structures and processes and indeed almost any kind of social or physical entity—may also be used in the service of symbolization. Mediation of man's knowledge of inner and outer reality by symbolic process is his unique characteristic, emerging at his level of biological organization. Symbolizing is as much a part of man's "biology" as the physiological processes constituting conditions and resources for symbolic process. "Biology" and "psychology" do not describe different empirical realms, and their separation as such has been decried, for example, by Heinz Hartmann [14, 15].

Man lives in symbolic reality partly because of the ambiguity of the object world and the plasticity of the nervous system [26]. By "ambiguity of the object world" we mean that the significance of an object for the goal-states the actor seeks in relation to it cannot be compelled by the object's intrinsic nature. The meaning of an object, of external reality, must be chosen by the actor from among possible alternatives; he may be said, thereby, to be making an interpretation of reality. Likewise, the plasticity of man's nervous system is its remarkable feature. The importance of fixed, predetermined stimulus-response mechanisms pales in comparison. Man's genetically given constitution does not determine a priori the nature of his intentions in a particular object-situation. The choice of what particular motivational dispositions are relevant, what meaning to give inner reality, also requires an act of interpretation.

The necessity of interpretation implies alternative frameworks of meaning, each characterized by a particular kind of symbolic process. To regard inner or outer reality in the terms of such a framework constitutes the act of interpretation determining what kind of reality is being created and the way in which it is experienced. The act of interpretation involves selecting, bringing to bear, or activating one framework of meaning from among a number of possible alternatives. The one chosen determines the form and organization of symbolic process—how the object, the actor, and the components of relationship between them will be symbolized.

Examples of frameworks of meaning, as these are given primacy in types of action or highly differentiated works of man are: the adaptive frame of reference exemplified in instrumental action and by science, with its concern with the relation of means to ends and its cognitive standards of truth, validity, or efficiency; the expressive frame of reference exemplified in expressive action and by art, with its representation of meanings by expressive symbolization and its appreciative or aesthetic standards of appropriateness, taste, or beauty; the moral frame of reference exemplified in responsible action and by law, with its moral evaluations in terms of systems of norms and its integrative standards of right and wrong; and the ideal frame of reference exemplified in commitments to patterns of ideals, values, and beliefs, and by religion, with its interest in maintaining patterns of beliefs about nonempirical aspects of reality and ultimate value-orientations. Similar formulations have been made by Cassirer and Parsons [4, 23].

Remembering earlier comments suggesting a contrast between psychic reality and "real" reality, I should like to reemphasize here that while "real" external reality may be presumed to exist independently of its apprehension, it cannot be known except symbolically—as part of psychic reality insofar as psychic reality is constituted by symbolic processes. Even the experience of "simple" sensations involves interpretation in a framework of meaning. Science, or an adaptive-cognitive orientation to reality, does not involve direct knowledge of "real" reality but an interpretation of reality in a particular framework of meaning. The achievement of science is its system of highly abstract cognitive representation of reality, to a great extent freed of particular sensuous connotations. However, science among the works of man and an adaptive-cognitive orientation to reality do not offer or lead to the only, or necessarily the best, interpretation of reality for all purposes or requirements of an individual or collective acting system. The utility of science, or an adaptive-cognitive orientation to reality, for the adaptive mastery of reality has tended to lead to its overvaluation in the behavioral sciences and to a concomitant lack of appreciation of other works of man and other orientations to reality as involving meaningful, functional frameworks of meaning within which acting systems may orient to and represent reality. Heinz Hartmann has made the similar point that rational action is not the only or always the best means of achieving an optimal relation between an acting system and its environment [14, 15].

What principles of organization of knowledge in the behavioral sciences follow from this view of man? Four empirical systems may be distinguished, each with its own characteristic boundaries, transactions across such boundaries, entities or component-units, and principles or rules of organization or of relationship between units. Each constitutes an analytically distinguishable empirical realm to the study of which unique concepts or variables, theories, and methods of investigation are relevant. The four systems are related to each other by a hierarchy of control in one direction and a hierarchy of constraint or conditions limiting possibility in the reverse direction. The following order of presentation is according to the hierarchy of control.

A *cultural system* is an organization of symbolic entities—such as values and beliefs, norms, expressive patterns, or adaptive-cognitive representations. Such symbolic patterns may be said to be institutionalized in a social system to the extent they are internalized by, and govern interactions between, members of the social system.

A *social system* is an organization of interacting social entities, performing in reciprocal, complementary roles, mutually regulated or integrated according to shared patterns of meaning. Role expectations become part of, shape, and modify the motivational dispositions of personality systems.

A *personality system* is an organization of motivational dispositions to achieve various kinds of ends. Such organizations of motivational dispositions control, activate, or determine the direction of expression or allocation of the resources and capacities of physiological behavioral organisms.

A *physiological behavioral organism* is an organization of physico-chemical entities, engaged in transactions across physical boundaries and resulting in capacities (also, facilities, media, opportunities, and occasions) and constraints, which essentially constitute the resources used in, and the conditions limiting, behavior [22, 23, 27].

It is this view of man and way of organizing knowledge in the behavioral sciences that has influenced our thinking about a behavioral sciences track curriculum.

COMPONENTS OF A BEHAVIORAL SCIENCES TRACK

The definition of the goal of such a track as the integration of the behavioral sciences and clinical experience implies that the track should include the following components.

1. There should be organized opportunities for *clinical experience.*

2. There should be formal seminars in the basic *behavioral sciences.* Such seminars might include a minimum core of courses especially prepared for the track as well as elective courses already existing in the medical school and university. (Presumably, each student will seek out particular electives to extend his knowledge in areas of special interest.)

3. There should be *mechanisms of integration,* the chief aim of which is to help the student to relate his clinical experience to his work in basic behavioral science. Such mechanisms might include special small group seminars in which current clinical experiences are presented and considered from the point of view of behavioral science knowledge, as well as a tutorial in which each student has a close, ongoing relationship with a member of the faculty. Ideally, both the student's research project and his clinical work in the track will place demands upon him to integrate clinical experience and behavioral science knowledge. At the same time the quality of the research project and clinical work will provide a test of the adequacy and extent of the integration the student has been able to achieve as a result of his participation in the track program.

Clinical Experience

As the program is presently planned, the medical student might spend up to five half-days a week acquiring clinical experience. One of these half-days will be spent in a general medicine outpatient clinic, an assignment which will be required of all medical students regardless of their individual tracks. A student might choose to spend, in addition, up to four half-days in clinical psychiatric settings.

The clinical experience in psychiatry should provide opportunities to study disease and recovery in physiological behavioral organisms, maladaptation and adaptation in personality systems, disorganization and reorganization in social systems, and incoherence and reformation in cultural systems.

There appear to be two possible strategies for organizing such clinical experience—each with advantages and disadvantages. Adopting one strategy, the medical student may elect to move from one setting to another. In each setting some particular empirical system might be clearly emphasized, confronting the student with typical differences in the kind of experience one has studying, or participating in, each such system. For example, the student might work one half-day on a neurology or endocrinology ward. In connection with this experience, work or demonstrations in a neurophysiological research laboratory might be provided. The student might work one half-day in an outpatient clinic doing individual psychotherapy. In connection with this experience, he might also elect to be in individual psychotherapy himself. He might work one half-day in an inpatient unit studying small group and organizational processes. In connection with this experience, he might also elect to be a member of a study group, where the task is both to participate in, and to study, small group processes as these occur. He might spend one half-day in a community, where the effects of the impact of one culture upon another and of cultural systems upon transactional processes are especially visible. For example, he might learn something about symbolic systems and their influence upon behavior by working in a "mixed" neighborhood, visiting a theater group in rehearsal, or studying the vicissitudes of personal counseling by representatives of different religious faiths. The disadvantages of such a strategy are the fragmentation of the student's clinical experience, the loss of continuous intensive participation in any particular process, and a possible emphasis on learning a variety of situation-specific techniques rather than an integrated approach to clinical phenomena.

Adopting another strategy, the student may elect to concentrate his clinical experience in *one* setting, changing his activities and conceptual focus within that setting. For example, he might participate on an inpatient unit or in a hospital organization: studying alterations in the neurophysiological functioning of particular patients; doing individual psychotherapy; conducting group therapy or participating in small group or intergroup meetings such as therapeutic community meetings; and observing the effects of different value, belief, and norm systems upon the behavior of members of the patient group and various professional staff groups both within such groups and in the contact of the members of such groups with each other. It might even be possible to try to understand a particular patient in these different ways, focusing now on aspects of his neurophysiological functioning, then on intrapsychic conflicts, now on his role behavior in various groups (such as the patient group or his own family group), and then on the characteristics of the symbolic forms, including language itself, which he has internalized or which impinge upon him in varying ways. The disadvantages of this strategy are difficulties, on the one hand, in finding clinical settings which offer a sufficient variety of experience and, on the other hand, in providing the student with conceptual tools rapidly enough for him to make such distinctions with respect to aspects of a particular phenomenon, or in recruiting clinical teachers possessing the requisite resources who can work closely enough with the student to stimulate him to focus in fact upon a specific phenomenon (for example, a particular patient) from the point of view of alternative frames of reference.

It is likely that the student will come to clinical experience in the track wanting to learn what to *do* in this or that situation, *to* this or that patient. "What is *the* treatment for 'schizophrenia'? What should I *do* when a patient 'acts out' in this way? What should I *say* when a patient says that? What is *the* technique for treating a mother and child; for treating a husband and wife; for treating a group of patients; for conducting a therapeutic community meeting? Which *one* is better, individual psychotherapy or community psychiatry?" The student's declared impatience with the academic; his quest for agents and gimmickry through which to bring about change; his apparent sense of himself as a computer processing objective data, a robot-like reactor to "the behaviors" of objects upon which he is to operate (as if "a behavior" were, in and of itself, an adequate, unambiguous sign), may easily parody a pseudotechnological ethos—"pseudo" because in such a state the value of active mastery through knowledge or understanding, which is the heart of technology, is absent.

Hopefully, the clinical teacher or supervisor in the track program will resist his students' demands for "practical answers" and insist instead upon formulating questions for which neither he nor the students have adequate answers. He will challenge his students' ways of thinking, and accept challenges to his own. He will share quandaries with his students, rather than facts and procedures. He will seek to enhance his students' skill, and by skill he will mean *not* facility of automatic manipulation in response to cues, but rather action that includes the ability to shift from one framework of meaning to another in the effort to understand many aspects of a complex phenomenon. Skill requires the ability to see an "illness," for example, in terms of neurophysiological structures and processes, which set the conditions and determine the availability of resources limiting functioning and thereby contribute to the shape of illness; in terms of an expressive symbolization of states on a continuum of gratification and deprivation of personal aims; again in terms of the role expectations in a system of interaction such as family or society that are met through the form illness takes; and even as in part a manifestation of a symbolic system of beliefs more or less private or shared with others.

It becomes increasingly clear that if such a track program is to succeed a new kind of clinical teacher is required; indeed, one of the first goals of the track program might have to be to help create such clinical teachers. The allegiance of such a teacher is not given exclusively to concepts or methods appropriate to the study of either physiological behavioral organism, personality system, social system, or cultural system as competing, mutually exclusive alternatives in the study of behavior. He is able to consider behavioral phenomena within the framework of any one of these systems, and, at the same time, in terms of the form of relationship between, or interarticulation of, such systems. The lack of such allegiance, as I have tried to show, is an expression not of aimless, uncommitted eclecticism, but rather of a certain view of man and the principles of organizing knowledge which follow from such a view.

If the clinical teacher succeeds, the student will turn with eager questions from his clinical experience in the track to the study of the basic behavioral sciences.

The Behavioral Sciences

What is the basic science knowledge applied in psychiatry? In the view presented here, it is the body of knowledge concerned with symbolic process, with man's symbolizing activities and achievements. More particularly, it is concerned with the conditions of, and resources for, symbolic processes in the physiological behavioral organism; with the symbolization of motivational dispositions and their fates in the personality system; with the integration of interacting entities according to shared patterns of meaning in the social system; and with the characteristics of cultural systems–symbolic forms (to use Cassirer's term [6]), organizations of symbolic entities, or works of man, such as language, myth, science, art, law, and religion, which may be institutionalized in social systems and internalized in personality systems.

Symbolic processes may go awry; aspects of symbolization may be impaired. Disorders in integration and adaptation of acting systems involve such impairment. Psychiatry, as one of the healing arts, may be regarded as the treatment–often, but by no means exclusively, through symbolic means–of "symbolic impairments." Robert Jay Lifton, for example, makes use of this term in the study, involving psychological, social, and cultural perspectives, of impairments of the symbolization of death [20]. Such impairments of symbolic process usually (but, given the limiting cases, not always) have origins, or are aggravated by processes, in all four systems–physiological behavioral organism, personality system, social system, and cultural system–and the complicated relationships among them. It is often difficult to know, with respect to a particular impairment of symbolization, to what system or relationship between systems treatment should be directed.

In the first two-and-a-half years of medical school, the student will have studied human development and psychopathology. Knowledge in these areas is assumed in planning the track. Four formal seminars in a basic behavioral sciences core curriculum will then be made available to the student during the first semester of the track: 1) The Physiological Behavioral Organism: Concepts and Methods; 2) The Personality System: Concepts and Methods; 3) The Social System: Concepts and Methods; and 4) The Cultural System: Concepts and Methods. Giving seminars on the four systems concurrently rather than serially or in different semesters is related to the intention to present the four systems as complementary perspectives, not as competing, mutually exclusive compartments of knowledge.

Four formal seminars in a basic behavioral sciences core curriculum will be made available to the student during the second semester of the track: 1) The Physiological Behavioral Organism: Stress and Adaptation, Disequilibrium and Homeostasis; 2) The Personality System: Conflict and Integration, Adaptation and Maladaptation; 3) The Social System: Disorganization and Control, Strain and Processes of Change; and 4) The Cultural System: Incoherence and Reformation, Patterns of Change.

One seminar in a basic behavioral sciences core curriculum will be offered during the third semester of the track: Relationships Between the Physiological Behavioral Organism, the Personality System, the Social System, and the Cultural System.

The first semester, then, focuses on problems of basic theory and research methodology in the study of the four behavioral science systems. The second semester focuses on processes of change as these occur in each of the four behavioral science systems. The third semester focuses on the integration of the behavioral sciences through the study of the relations between—the inputs and outputs across the boundaries of—the four behavioral science systems. The integration of behavioral science and clinical experience within the student is manifested by skill; the integration of the behavioral sciences themselves is manifested by conceptual clarity.

The time allocated to seminars in the basic behavioral sciences core curriculum should probably decrease from the first to the second semester by about fifty percent, and from the second to the third semester by another fifty percent, with the expectation that over the three semesters a student will devote himself increasingly to his individual research project and to electives related to his specialized area of interest. Ordinarily, within such limits, the members and teachers of each seminar will have the freedom to decide together about frequency of meeting and length of session.

Three strategies concerning the basic behavioral sciences core curriculum have been tentatively adopted:

1. In this part of the track program, basic behavioral science knowledge will be presented, rather than the studies sometimes referred to as "behavioral science" that are actually applications

of behavioral science knowledge to clinical psychiatric problems. The application of behavioral science will be the main theme of the third component of the track (to be discussed below), which is devoted to mechanisms of integrating behavioral science with clinical experience. The goal of the basic behavioral sciences core curriculum is achievement by the student of four different perspectives on human behavior—an ability to understand phenomena from the point of view of any of the four systems we have been describing, and recognition of what is unique to, and characteristic of, each view. The student, as an outcome of his participation in the track, should be able, for example, to study psychological phenomena as constituting an empirical system in its own right, without reduction of personality to physiology, and a social system as a social system, not as a mere summation or expression of individual motives, nor as a kind of personality system on a large scale.

2. The seminars in the basic behavioral sciences core curriculum will be conducted at a graduate level. The method of choice will be the intensive study and group discussion of a few classical monographs in each seminar, rather than lectures and long reading lists aiming at an overview of a congeries of miscellaneous data. By a classical monograph we mean a work illustrating, when possible, both methodological problems of empirical research and a strategy of theory formation and its consequences, with justice given to the complexity of these problems in studying a particular behavioral science system. What we shall eschew especially is the oversimplification that is attractive because it is easily assimilable. Where there is a choice between a monograph or paper that confines itself to theory, analysis of methodological issues, or description of empirical data, and a monograph or paper involving empirical research explicitly and meaningfully related to theory, we would select the latter. It is expected, of course, that the group discussion of the theoretical, methodological, and substantive issues raised by the intensive study of such classical monographs will stimulate the student to read on his own a variety of related, complementary or controverting works, which will, of course, be referred to in discussion.

Everyone will have his own preferences in selecting such monographs; the following list is suggestive rather than prescriptive.

The first semester seminars emphasizing concepts and methods might focus upon such classical works as Cannon's *Wisdom of the Body* [3], Freud's *The Interpretation of Dreams* [11], Parsons' *The Social System* [24], and Cassirer's studies of symbolic forms such as language, myth, and scientific thought [4, 5, 6].

Other works that might be considered in the first seminar are Cannon's *Bodily Changes in Pain, Hunger, Fear, and Rage,* Gardner, et al, *Cognitive Control: A Study of Individual Consistencies in Cognitive Behavior,* Hebb's *Organization of Behavior,* Heider's *On Perception, Event Structure, and the Psychological Environment,* the body of research concerned with sleep and dreaming, or studies of brain structure and chemistry, and psychological function; in the second seminar, Freud's *The Psychopathology of Everyday Life, Jokes and Their Relation to the Unconscious, Three Essays on the Theory of Sexuality,* and *Two Principles of Mental Functioning,* or another group of writings about personality by Lewin and Tolman, with their emphasis on goal-orientation in terms of "life space" or "cognitive map;" in the third seminar, Durkheim's *Division of Labor in Society,* Durkheim's *The Elementary Forms of Religious Life,* Etzioni's *A Comparative Analysis of Complex Organizations,* papers from Hare's collection of studies *Small Groups,* Lynd and Lynd's *Middletown: A Study in Contemporary Culture,* Parsons' *Structure of Social Action,* Weber's *The Sociology of Religion,* Weber's *Theory of Economic and Social Organization,* or Whyte's *Street Corner Society;* and in the fourth seminar, Benedict's *Patterns of Culture,* Kenneth Burke's *Permanence and Change, Grammar of Motives, Rhetoric of Motives,* and his studies of symbolic action, Langer's *Philosophy in a New Key,* Piaget's studies, with emphasis on his investigation of different modes of cognition and moral evaluation rather than on developmental issues per se, Whorf's *Science and Linguistics,* or Zborowski and Herzog's *Life Is With People.*

The second semester seminars emphasizing processes of change might focus upon such classical works as Selye's research on stress and adaptation [30], Freud's *Studies in Hysteria* and case histories [11], Durkheim's *Suicide* [7], and Sorokin's *Social and Cultural Dynamics* [32].

These works might be supplemented in the first seminar by the body of research concerned with sensory deprivation; studies of the relation between structural lesions, toxic conditions, or aberrant brain biochemistry, and such symbolic functions as use of language or consciousness; in the second seminar by Freud's papers on neurosis and psychosis; in the third seminar by Becker's *Outsiders: Studies in the Sociology of Deviance,* Jaques' *The Changing Culture of a Factory,* Rice's *The Enterprise and its Environment,* and Sofer's *The Organization from Within*—these three describing attempts to bring about change in organizations, papers from Hare's collection of studies *Small Groups,* Lewin's *Resolving Social Conflicts,* Smelser's *Theory of Collective Behavior*—an attempt to account for panics, crazes and fads, hostile outbursts, and social movements; and in the fourth seminar by Lynd and Lynd's *Middletown in Transition: A Study in Cultural Conflicts.*

In the third semester seminar, concerned with the integration of, or relations between, the four behavioral science systems, two approaches are possible. In one, a particular system may be chosen as focal, and inputs to this system from the other systems (as well as outputs from this system to the other systems) may be studied. For example, the personality system may be chosen as focal, and inputs from the physiological behavioral organism, the social system, and the cultural system may then be examined, as approximated in the organization of Kluckhohn and Murray's collection of studies, *Personality in Nature, Society, and Culture* [17]. Erikson's work is apposite here [10].

In a second approach, two systems may be studied in relation to each other, as interarticulated in some crucial way, or according to an independent-dependent variable or interacting variable paradigm—as in Smelser and Smelser's collection of studies, *Personality and Social Systems* [31], or such a work as Weber's *The Protestant Ethic and the Spirit of Capitalism* [35] in which cultural systems of religious values and beliefs are related to social structure. Other works that might be included here are Freud's

Group Psychology and the Analysis of the Ego, Kardiner's *The Individual and His Society* and *The Psychological Frontiers of Society,* some of the works of Kurt Lewin and his followers, Merton's *Bureaucratic Structure and Personality,* and Parsons' *Social Structure and Personality.* At least three sets of system pairs could be studied in this way: physiological behavioral organism and personality system; personality system and social system; social system and cultural system.

3. The third and final strategy concerning the basic behavioral sciences core curriculum is reflected in our hope that a basic behavioral scientist and clinical psychiatrist will conduct each seminar in the curriculum together. This hope comes from our recognition of the medical student's hunger for models with whom to identify, and his tendency to reject nonclinical and especially nonphysician teachers as irrelevant or inappropriate to his purposes, unless there is an obvious alliance between such teachers and the clinical teacher, who is interested in, respects, and makes use of their work. It also comes from our judgment that the integration of behavioral science knowledge and clinical experience requires that the teacher conducting a seminar devoted to that task has participated in the basic science seminars and will be able to demonstrate the relevance of such knowledge for clinical practice. The plan, then, is that the clinical psychiatrist member of the teaching teams in the basic science seminars will take major responsibility for a seminar concerned with the integration of basic science and clinical experience.

Mechanisms of Integration

The major mechanism of integration in the track program, in addition to the tutorial previously mentioned, will be a seminar tentatively entitled *OII: Observation, Interpretation, and Integration* after a famous course in the liberal arts college of the University of Chicago. OII will probably meet, as a small group or in small group sections, once a week throughout the three semesters of the track. The principal theme of the seminar will be "problems of treatment." A typical discussion might proceed as follows.

1. A student may present observations from his clinical experience in any one of a variety of situations in which he has had responsibility for skillful intervention.

2. Members of the group may then discuss: "How might such phenomena be interpreted? What frames of reference might be brought to bear? How may we understand these phenomena in terms of what we are learning about the physiological behavioral organism, the personality system, the social system, the cultural system?" It is in this part of the discussion that the group may consult research and other writings concerned with the application of behavioral science knowledge to clinical-psychiatric problems.

3. The discussion may conclude with the implications of such interpretations for skillful intervention—that is, with some attempt at an integration of knowledge with experience resulting in the possibility of skillful intervention.

Suppose, for example, a student presents observations from a situation in which he was concerned with the treatment of a so-called schizophrenic patient. The various perspectives used in interpretation of the phenomena in group discussion may lead to interest in the following kinds of questions:

1. What values concerning health, illness, and treatment and what beliefs about "schizophrenia" guide the action of the physician who attempts to treat a patient who has been designated by a symbol such as "schizophrenic"? How coherent are such systems of values and beliefs: what contradictions do they contain? What attempts are made by the physician to accommodate, or defend against, such contradictions? The same questions may be asked about any members of the allied professions involved in such treatment, about the student himself, and also about the patient's own attitudes toward health, illness, and treatment, as well as his particular illness, as these attitudes affect his own participation in the treatment endeavor. Parsons' analysis of the case of modern medical practice is relevant here [24].

2. What normative expectations define the roles and role relationships of the physician, members of allied professions, and the patient? What inconsistencies exist in such expectations? What

accommodations are made to such inconsistencies? What are the functional and dysfunctional consequences of a particular set of role definitions [9, 18]? How do individual personalities make use of roles to defend against anxiety or to gratify idiosyncratic aims [21]?

3. What are the characteristics of the situational context in which treatment is attempted, and how are these characteristics reflected in the vicissitudes of the treatment process? The situation includes the hospital or other organizational settings as well as the extended community involving a social class structure and a variety of reference groups, both formal and primary, to which the physician, members of allied professions, student, and patient are in relation [8, 9, 13, 16, 33]. Here, for example, the group may consider how a schizophrenic patient's suicidal act is an outcome not only of intrapsychic processes but of group processes on an inpatient unit leading to the commitment of a series of such acts by different individuals.

4. How is the illness itself to be understood? What contributes to the etiology of schizophrenia, from the point of view taken: in genetic and biochemical research; in the study of the personality system of the schizophrenic patient as carried out, for example, in intensive individual psychotherapy; in the investigations of disordered transactions in families of patients with schizophrenia [19]; in the investigations of schizophrenia in different cultures and different strata of a particular society; and in the investigations of the relation of personal disorganization to community disorganization?

5. Finally, the group may turn to the question of treatment interventions. Toward what change in what system or systems should such interventions be directed? What does the choice of a locus of intervention imply for the kinds of skill required to help make such change possible? What, for example, is the distinction between sociotherapy and psychotherapy with reference to the system of concern, and between the skills required by the psychotherapist and sociotherapist [9]?

Clearly, having available an indexed collection of applications of behavioral science to clinical-psychiatric problems—classified according to such topics as "values and beliefs," "roles," "situational context," and "illness"–would be of great help to such a seminar group. At least one selected bibliography without special reference to clinical-psychiatric problems but for medical behavioral science in general, with titles classified according to such topics as "roles and role relations," "structural and organizational context of therapy," and "clinical problems," is in existence [28].

CONCLUSION

This, then, is our vision of what a behavioral sciences track might be like, unaltered by mundane considerations of such constraints as available resources (for example, money, meeting space, clinical facilities, books and journals, and personnel with requisite teaching skills and knowledge), the motivational states of medical students, the motivational states of faculty members, the impact of competing conceptions, and emerging requirements for administrative accommodation to other track programs. How such constraints will alter the shape of the behavioral sciences track as vision becomes actuality remains to be discovered.

REFERENCES

Note: The thinking about and planning for a behavioral sciences track in the medical school curriculum reported in this chapter developed in discussions with the members of the track subcommittee of the undergraduate training committee of the department of psychiatry, Yale University (Kenneth Keniston, Ph.D., Braxton McKee, M.D., Michael Sheard, M.D., and Harvey Wasserman, M.D.), and with Theodore Lidz, M.D., while the author was chairman of that subcommittee.

1. Bertalanffy, L. von. 1968. *Organismic psychology and systems theory.* Worcester: Clark University Press.
2. Burke, K. 1964. *Perspectives by incongruity.* Bloomington: Indiana University Press.
3. Cannon, W. 1932. *The wisdom of the body.* New York: W. W. Norton.
4. Cassirer, E. 1944. *An essay on man.* New Haven: Yale University Press.
5. ——. 1953. *Language and myth.* New York: Dover Publications.

6. ——. 1953. *The philosophy of symbolic forms.* New Haven: Yale University Press.
7. Durkheim, E. 1951. *Suicide.* Glencoe: The Free Press.
8. Edelson, M. *Group life in a psychiatric hospital.* In preparation.
9. ——. 1970. *Sociotherapy and psychotherapy.* Chicago: University of Chicago Press.
10. Erikson, E. 1950. *Childhood and society.* New York: W. W. Norton.
11. Freud, S. 1953. *The standard edition of the complete psychological works of Sigmund Freud.* London: Hogarth Press.
12. GAP Report No. 42. 1959. Some observations on controls in psychiatric research.
13. Greenblatt, M., et al, eds. 1957. *The patient and the mental hospital.* Glencoe: The Free Press.
14. Hartman, H. 1958. *Ego psychology and the problem of adaptation.* New York: International Universities Press.
15. Hartman, H. 1964. *Essays on ego psychology.* New York: International Universities Press.
16. Hollingshead, A. B., and Redlich, F. C. 1958. *Social class and mental illness.* New York: John Wiley.
17. Kluckhohn, C. K., and Murray, H. A., eds. 1949. *Personality in nature, society, and culture.* New York: Alfred A. Knopf.
18. Levinson, D. S., and Gallagher, B. 1964. *Patienthood in the mental hospital.* Boston: Houghton Mifflin.
19. Lidz, T., Fleck, S., and Cornelison, A. 1965. *Schizophrenia and the family.* New York: International Universities Press.
20. Lifton, R. J. 1968. *Death in life: survivors of Hiroshima.* New York: Random House.
21. Menzies, I. 1960. A case-study in the functioning of social systems as a defence against anxiety: a report on a study of the nursing service of a general hospital. *Human Relations* 13:95-121.
22. Parsons, T. 1959. An approach to psychological theory in terms of the theory of action. In *Psychology: a science,* vol. 3, ed. S. Koch. New York: McGraw-Hill.
23. ——. 1960. Pattern variables revisited. *American Sociological Review* 25, no. 4 (August).
24. ——. 1951. *The social system.* New York: The Free Press of Glencoe.
25. ——. 1949. *The structure of social action.* 2d ed. New York: The Free Press of Glencoe.
26. ——, and Shils, E., eds. 1951. *Toward a general theory of action.* New York: Harper and Row (Torchbook Edition, 1962).
27. ——, et al, eds. 1961. *Theories of society,* 2 vols. New York: The Free Press of Glencoe.
28. Pearsall, M. 1963. *Medical behavioral science: a selected bibliography of cultural anthropology, social psychology, and sociology in medicine.* Lexington, Ky.: University of Kentucky Press.
29. Rice, A. K. 1963. *The enterprise and its environment.* London: Tavistock Publications.

30. Selye, H. 1952. *The story of the adaptation syndrome.* Montreal: Acta Medical Publications.
31. Smelser, N. J., and Smelser, W. T. 1963. *Personality and social systems.* New York: John Wiley and Sons.
32. Sorokin, P. 1937-40. *Social and cultural dynamics,* 4 vols. New York: American Book.
33. Stanton, A. H., and Schwartz, M. S. 1954. *The mental hospital.* New York: Basic Books.
34. Stone, L. 1961. *The psychoanalytic situation.* New York: International Universities Press, Inc.
35. Weber, M. 1930. *The protestant ethic and the spirit of capitalism.* London: Allen and Unwin.

3. The "Mixed Psychiatry/Medicine" Internship Program of the Upstate Medical Center

Donald Oken, M.D.

It is a great pleasure to write about our "mixed psychiatry/medicine" internship program at Syracuse. For one thing, we are proud of it. Moreover, a consideration of some of the underlying issues which are involved will, I think, be instructive. Certainly we have learned a lot from it.

This innovative program was a product of the imagination, courage, and foresight of Dr. Marc Hollender, then chairman of the department of psychiatry at Upstate. As a matter of fact, I have had only about six months of direct experience with the program. This puts me in that delightful position in which, not burdened by undue familiarity, I can provide you with a report uncluttered by many facts! Perhaps, however, there is some advantage to my state of relative ignorance. It allows me the vantage point of an outside observer who has not developed an over-identification with the program, but who nevertheless has some of the insider's knowledge.

In any event, I do not expect to provide you with a description of the minute details of the program. Rather, I intend primarily to examine the rationale of the program from a more conceptual viewpoint, doing so against the broader background of the purposes and goals of internship generally.

You will recall that this program was established in 1960. As described then by Dr. Hollender [4], its basic outlines are:

> The intern spends six months each on psychiatry and on medicine. During the period on psychiatry, he functions much as a junior resident does, in that he is responsible for evaluating and treating hospitalized patients. He receives individual supervision and participates in conferences. Selected seminars are open to him.

It should be added that one month within the period assigned to medicine is spent on the neurological service, during which the interns' duties are arranged to emphasize the more relevant aspects of that field.

The key phrase in the description is "he functions much as a junior resident does." As a matter of fact, we can now state more accurately that he functions *as* a junior resident–we make no distinctions between these interns and our first year residents. Except for the time span, they have identical clinical assignments and equal responsibility for patients, and they attend the same courses and conferences.

As Marc Hollender also noted [4], the design of this program represented an attempt to take a "halfway position" on two fundamental issues in medical education. The first is concerned with the overall necessity of an internship within the already prolonged period of education, and the second with the necessity for a psychiatrist to be grounded in clinical medicine. His perspicacity in not only recognizing the importance of these issues but being responsive to them at so early a date is impressive. At the present time they have gained major importance and constitute a central focus of dialogue among medical educators.

There is, however, a bit of irony here. I think it an accurate interpretation of the situation in 1960 to characterize as courageous and progressive the enacting of a program which embodied even a compromise between the polar responses to these two questions. In those days, a move away from the year of internship and any question of the notion that a psychiatrist must first be a *medical* doctor met with widespread resistance, if not rage. Now, however, I read the winds of change differently. Although still in process, the forces operating in the direction of abolishing internships and substituting a year representing an earlier start on residency training are growing to be preeminent; and the defender of the mixed internship may be cast in the role of an arch-conservative. I am afraid I am going to have to take that risk–though my own view is that this position has more gold in it than Goldwater.

As a psychiatrist, my approach is, properly, dynamic and genetic. The primary questions are motivational: What are the purposes, goals or functions of an internship? These questions are best scrutinized from the developmental standpoint: How are their current expressions related to the past?

In this country, medical training began almost entirely as individual apprenticeship focusing on the acquisition of skills of the trade. There was minimum basic science, save for a little anatomy, and no concept of medicine as an applied science. Then medical schools, which had developed slowly at first, began to burgeon. A few attempted to teach what was known of the basic sciences, though they primarily transmitted the knowledge which was being acquired in the laboratories of flourishing European medical centers. Not all made that effort, however; many were mere diploma mills. Under the housecleaning impact of the Flexner Report [2], the latter group were forced into oblivion. The character of American medical education thus was almost completely reversed from its beginnings. Now it was conceived as a period of academic education based on the knowledge and principles of science. With this transformation, however, came the new and opposite consequence of producing physicians who had never had any real experience in treating sick people. (The danger of any cleanup is that, carried far enough, it may yield total sterility.)

In response to this deficiency, two correctives were developed. One was the inclusion of clinical experience within the undergraduate medical curriculum. The other, initially of much greater significance, was the decision to append a period of formal graduate medical education, the internship. As originally conceived, the internship represented a revival of apprenticeship as a method for acquiring the skills of practice, albeit in a new fashion which embodied quality control. Growing sophistication, however, began to make it clear that the apprenticeship model would not do. The passive acquisition of facts and their utilization via modeling on the pattern provided by one's seniors proved to be inadequate. It was recognized that an internship should represent instead a period of graded clinical experience, providing the opportunity for *self*-education, augmented by teaching. The basic design of the internship was, of course, "rotating" in type, planned to provide the necessary breadth of exposure for future (general) practitioners. Although this was for some time quite satisfactory, the forces of change made it necessary to modify that design. The forces I refer to include the explosion in the quantity of scientific knowledge, the increasing development and application of technological advances, the progressive development of and emphasis on specialization, and the revolution in many parts of our social order. All have been profoundly important as trends in their own right as well as in their complex interrelationships [1, 7]. But all had the same effect: pushing the internship toward greater concentration on fewer, more specialized fields.

In addition, there was a problem inherent within the rotating concept itself. The usual rotation had much the quality of a whirling revolving door, providing breadth of exposure at the expense of depth. The intern was exposed to a series of stroboscopic images of patients and separate specialties. This sharply limited his opportunity to acquire a genuinely integrated knowledge of medicine, or of whole patients. Hence it became necessary to provide rotations which involved spending greater periods of time on fewer, major services. The extension of this principle (along with the effects of the other change factors noted) led to the concept of the "mixed" internship, with assignments limited to two, three, or perhaps four services, and to the straight internship restricted to one service.

The same forces have also served as major influences on the medical school curriculum. In the immediate post-Flexner era, clinical teaching within the medical school was extremely limited. Predominant reliance was placed upon didactic presentations and demonstrations, and these were concentrated in the later years. Over time, both the amount and scope of this experience has been broadened. Now, from their very first days, our students are provided with didactic teaching and applied problems involving the correlation of clinical issues with the basic sciences, and they have early direct patient contact which involves at least some—and in many instances major—personal clinical responsibility, under appropriate supervision. The traditional division into "preclinical" and "clinical" years has become almost meaningless. Moreover, in recent times specialization has entered significantly as a characteristic within the undergraduate years too. This has evolved via such mechanisms as provision for major time segments in which students elect their courses (which may occupy the entire fourth year and more) or the early selection of one of a series of "tracks" of course work.

These changes in the direction of greater clinical experience, which I view as highly salutary, have usurped many of the functions of the traditional internship. Today's students have more and better opportunities for acquiring clinical knowledge through experience than did many interns in the past. Simultaneously, the development of residencies has put heavy pressure on the internship from above. The overwhelming majority of physicians now engage in such specialty training [1]. Given the immense and expanding quantity of learning now required for mastery of a specialty and the practical limitation of time, the once shocking question of abolishing the hallowed internship is now voiced freely [7].

In one sense, straight (and mixed) internships have represented a way of begging that question. Many would contend that the straight internship is often, in effect, an extra residency year, called by another name to retain its sweetness for those who cannot bear so radical a challenge to their rosy evaluation of the status quo. That such a view is at least partly correct seems irrefutable. However, even where that is so, there appears to be a highly significant difference between that first year and the subsequent residency. This difference rests on the relative distinction between what I would term general and special education (obviously I do not mean here education for the practice of general medicine). The residency concentrates on the acquisition of knowledge and effective skills in that specialty via care for patients, whereas the internship focuses more on learning how to be effective with patients via work in that specialty.

In terms of this distinction, the validity of retaining the internship year rests, of course, on whether that "general" learning can occur just as well either prior to it or afterwards, i.e. in medical school or during residency. At least two major determinants are involved in this: the specialty area and the structural characteristics of the training program. Among the factors involved in the latter are the nature of the house officer-patient relationships and the rotational features of the service. On most inpatient services it is the intern who sees the patient first—when he is most distressed; and on a day-to-day basis it is the intern who carries out the ongoing care. In sum, he acts as the patient's *physician*. If, however, the intern shifts from ward to ward too frequently, this effect is diluted. Too often he will arrive or leave in the middle of the patient's illness, and thus he functions as a mere interchangeable component within a computerized model of medical care. Under such an arrangement the intern not only will acquire that destructive self-concept but will have great difficulty even in learning to be a physician, as separate from being merely the holder of an M.D. degree.

It is perfectly obvious that it is the nature of the first-year house officer's functions which matters, not his title. He can as well be called a junior resident as an intern as long as his experience is along the lines I have described. Indeed there is an advantage to his being in the first year of an ongoing series constituting a residency, since that lends itself to orderly, overall continuity of programming for his entire period of formal postgraduate training. The value of this has been emphasized recently by both the Coggeshall [1] and Millis [7] reports.

What also matters is *which specialty* we are considering. Let me remind you that current 'straight' internships are confined (with rare exceptions such as pathology where the internship might better be conceived of as a fellowship) to the fields of internal medicine, general surgery and pediatrics. Internships in such fields as neurology, dermatology, orthopedics, G.U., or ENT are *not* considered acceptable. As a matter of fact, for the surgical specialties, many authorities consider a year of general surgical training to be a prerequisite for—indeed a part of—adequate training. The crucial question arises, then, whether psychiatry is sufficiently different from these other specialties as not to require some equivalent of grounding in medicine.

Before we examine this question, let us take a deeper look at the functions which an internship now serves. The traditional view would emphasize the acquisition of facts and skills. Our more sophisticated view would modify this with emphasis instead upon learning how to integrate data, how to reason, and how to apply knowledge in clinical problem solving. But even this updated version of the learning function may well be covered adequately by medical school clerkships, as I indicated earlier, although we must be cautious in assuming that this is a ubiquitous phenomenon. The statement that students now learn more clinical medicine than did past interns is deceptive. The real question is whether they learn enough in terms of the demands of *today's* clinical demands.

Obviously, we need to look further. Here, I would suggest that at least two other functions of greater significance are served by the internship. One concerns the socialization of the student into the role of the physician [6]: the acquisition of those attitudes, sets, and behavior styles–apart from technical knowledge on the one hand and individual psychological characteristics on the other–which characterize a doctor *qua* doctor. These include his ways of behavior and thought in relating to patients, colleagues, and allied health workers and, most significantly, his conception of *himself* in these relationships. Earlier I made essentially the same point, from another perspective, in pointing out the value of the internship for learning the skills of patient care, grounded in the continuing responsibility for and close relation to patients involved. Here I am emphasizing the *role* learning, which requires both the private and public recognition of the definition of an intern as doctor. It is because of this role definition that a medical student is not simply a less completely educated doctor who happens to lack his degree. One is reminded of the almost ubiquitous phenomenon of "graduation jitters" experienced by students in anticipation of their internship responsibilities. In spite of their intensive clinical experience, the validation of the responsibility they will be expected to shoulder as "doctors" leads to an entirely different subjective experience.

Of course the resident too is cast in the doctor's role. But his opportunities for learning this role are different because of the different role functions which a "specialist" assumes, and given the increasing tendency for specialization within medical school, one wonders if there will be any point other than the internship for learning the general role of the physician. To a significant extent, the specialist focuses on an organ or organ system, not the organism. (One has only to scan any typical history written by, say, an ENT resident to confirm this: I think it is safe to say that this is true on almost all specialty services.) The notable exceptions to this generalization are, of course, internal medicine and, perhaps to a lesser extent, general surgery. In these fields, the first year trainee, be he called intern or resident, learns what it is to be a physician in the generic sense. It is precisely this fact which, in my view, constitutes the basis for accepting a year in these specialties as the initial period of training for other fields, since they provide the "general" learning function which I have described.

The key question thus arises as to whether we can conclude the same thing about the psychiatric residency. Given our repeated (and pious) statements that psychiatry is par excellence the field interested in "the whole man" one might be inclined to think it is. I trust I will not be considered as a cynic in indicating grave doubts on this score. Most of our residency training activities are, to my view, weighted in the direction of preoccupation with the psychological, attenuated by some concern for the social. (At some places, in these days of preoccupation with community psychiatry and social action, the two emphases may be reversed.) But they do not for the most part evince an adequate awareness of the biological, including both the basic bio-behavioral sciences and especially the other (i.e. nonpsychiatric) clinical sciences. Nor do they integrate these into a total approach. We do provide great breadth of didactic training, but this is undermined by the nature of the clinical activities and the supervision thereon. For example, it is far from uncommon for the physical examination on a psychiatric service to be performed by medical interns or residents assigned there. While I may be mildly overstating the point, and the situation may be improving, I think it is an accurate one. In general, psychiatric residents tend to establish somewhat skewed doctor-patient relationships in which they are concerned largely with psychodynamic issues. Even clinical psychopathology suffers by contrast [3]. While this imbalance might be appropriate for the trained specialist, I do not see it as providing the breadth of experience that will allow the first-year-level *trainee* to develop his fundamental appreciation of the total patient. Hence, I do not feel the psychiatric residency can adequately supplant the internship.

That conclusion may be arguable, and I suspect it may raise some heat. But there is an additional function served by the internship which I find even harder to conceive as being fulfilled by the psychiatric residency. This I term its "tempering" function, analogous to the process of perfecting steel which is at once hard and resilient. The intern is exposed directly to situations of major emergency in which his actions *literally* mean the difference between life and death. Of necessity he learns how to respond rapidly, establish action priorities, and exercise judgment "under fire." At the same time that he experiences miraculous cures, he learns that some patients—some of *his* patients—die, despite his every effort. He learns how to work, and work well, in the face of personal exhaustion. I would suggest that out of these unpleasant and arduous experiences derives an orientation toward human beings in distress, and toward responsibility to them, that can be obtained so well in no other way. This is not to romanticize the internship as a drama nor to rationalize the exploitation of interns. But it is to recognize the poignant significance inherent in the literality of the life and death responsibilities involved. I would submit that psychiatry is one of those specialties where this quality is sufficiently attenuated as to fail to provide this function adequately. I do not say it does not occur at all, but only not as well nor as much as it should.

I happen to be one of those "traitors to my class" who feel strongly that a clinical psychologist has every bit as much right to become a psychotherapist as does a psychiatrist. But one problem which I (and my colleagues) have noted repeatedly as psychotherapy supervisors is a serious difficulty in the acquisition by psychology trainees of the nature of a therapist's commitment to a patient, especially one with more pervasive psychopathology. In no way am I implying that these trainees are irresponsible; indeed at times they tend to take on themselves too much of a sense of responsibility. What I refer to is the quality, not the extent of their sense of responsibility. It would not be germane to pursue the more complex issue of the distinctive roles which a psychiatrist and a psychologist can serve. But I would mention that the absence of the "tempering experience" also serves as a serious impediment in the eventual function of the psychiatrist as a consultant to other physicians. It leaves him with a lack of adequate appreciation for the experience both of the doctor and the patient.

By now, it must be clear why I see a period of postgraduate experience in clinical medicine as an essential feature of psychiatric training. At the same time I am cognizant of the reasons why we must try to keep this period to a minimum. Some of these I indicated earlier. If I have failed to highlight them adequately here, it is only because I feel less need to focus on them at this point in the history of medical education.

The mixed psychiatry/medicine internship as it has been pioneered at Syracuse, represents one solution to this dilemma. This program represents for us a compromise genuinely responsive to the essential aspects of both issues, not a mere expedient designed to satisfy progress while placating traditions or straddle an issue too controversial to face.

Having pontificated at some length—hopefully not in the form of a bull—let me now give you some concrete information about our program. For the first two years after it began in 1960, positions were opened only to our own Upstate Medical Center graduates. Again to quote Marc Hollender [5], "Although we believed that the internship would prove workable and worthwhile, we were inclined to move slowly and cautiously. When our expectations were matched by experience, we enlarged the program [initially to four interns] and opened it to outside applicants."

From that time, the internship has had a substantial number of applicants, never less than twice the number of available positions and more often three to four times that number. (This year, for example, we received fifty-three inquiries and wound up submitting twenty-four names in our ranking for the ten positions we made available.) By general standards of intelligence and maturity, this group has been superior on the average to our straight medical interns who enter psychiatry. They have been a superior group also when considered from the special standpoint of their potential as psychiatrists. In this regard, they are better than the pool of those who apply for our residency (though not necessarily better than those whom we have *selected*). Generally they are independent thinkers, well read, highly motivated for work in psychiatry, and psychologically minded and socially conscious. They are sophisticated about the field, as illustrated by their very awareness of the existence of our special program. This inference is supported by the fact that they are by no means all from nearby medical schools. Rather, they are fairly representative in geographical distribution of the national sample of residency applicants. Although our own students constitute the largest single group, they are far from a majority. The thirty-four past and current interns represent sixteen medical schools in addition to our own. These are somewhat predominantly in the Northeast, but not in greater proportion than the number of schools in this area. All but four of the interns have been male—the ladies have been selected only in the past two years, a phenomenon for which I have no explanation (but which I certainly intend to perpetuate!). Their age is about that of the usual intern, and correspondingly, the number who have previously had graduate training in some related field is not greater than what we see in our residents.

A prime question that must have arisen by now is the one of recruiting: Is this program a way of attracting residents to our program? I confess that I might be somewhat loath to reveal this if it were so. However I am relieved of a need to dissimulate as I see no real evidence for drawing such a conclusion. The number of our graduates who have gone on to other centers is essentially the same as those who enter the internship from outside, though these are not necessarily the same individuals. They have gone to a somewhat smaller number of *programs* than those they come from: twelve outside our own. (If I may say so, this reflects a predominant concentration at the better training centers, though I carefully refrain from suggesting just which I feel these are.) Some are attracted to stay at Upstate but others have indicated that having spent a year here and learned something of the special things we have to offer, they now specifically want to go elsewhere for a broader perspective—and many come with that in mind. As I have said, this is a sophisticated, independent group.

I think it is evident also that we have not recruited anyone additional into the field of psychiatry, though sometimes we may have helped to crystallize and confirm this career line. The applicants are a self-selected group of future psychiatrists. At the time of its inception, it was thought that this program would be attractive and helpful to selected future internists and pediatricians. By this criterion the internship can be regarded as *not* successful. Dr. Hollender [5] indicated that only four of fifty applicants as of 1964 had primary motivations to enter other fields. Thus far every single graduate has gone on to a psychiatric residency although not always in direct linear progression. (A current intern —one of those aberrant females!—has decided on a dermatology residency; it will be of interest to see if she stays in that field.) However, as already indicated, this is a function of their self-selection rather than our influence. It is always possible that our subtle biases operated in this direction at the time of our decisions of whom to accept, but our impression is that essentially all of our applicants had by then already decided upon a career in psychiatry. In any event, based on our experience, it is clear why I have limited my discussion of our mixed internship to its place in *psychiatric* education and have not compared it to other innovative mixed or rotating programs with different objectives.

Based on the criterion of customer satisfaction, the program has been a great success. Our interns come with the expectation that they can begin significant psychiatric training earlier by a half a year and "waste" correspondingly less time on less relevant activities (i.e. internal medicine). They have finished with that expectation satisfied. The most significant element in this is the fact, already stressed, that they are, operationally, first year residents while on the six-month assignment to psychiatry. They have relished their clearly defined responsibility for patients and full participation in our departmental teaching activities at that level [5].

From our perspective as faculty, we are equally satisfied. Our colleagues in medicine tell us that these have been good interns on their service—better, interestingly, than the average straight intern who plans on a career in psychiatry. As interns on psychiatry they have functioned as well as beginning residents. For whatever it is worth as validation of the effectiveness of their medical training, every one of the graduating interns, so far as we know, has passed Part III National Boards on the first try. When they become residents at Upstate they have been judged to be excellent, and reports from other residency centers to which they have migrated are similarly enthusiastic. Our graduates have gone on to what we feel are, for the most part, quite significant activities. For example, of the nine relatively recent graduates known to be in military service, four have been working at NIMH. A very large proportion of those who have reached the point of practicing psychiatry have entered upon academic careers, although they seem to have no special tendency to focus primarily on research activity despite some such hopes expressed at the time the program was begun. We must be cautious, however, in drawing conclusions from these data. We can say the program has been a great success, but we cannot say that this is entirely due to its inherent characteristics. There is no way to distinguish the merits of the program itself from the assets which this special pool of exciting young people bring to it.

The program is a success judged also by the evidence of national popularity. As I have indicated, the number of positions we have offered has increased from two to ten. Since the high ratio of applicants has remained relatively stable in the face of this growth—and increasing outside competition—the program seems to meet a need. The outside competition, in providing the sincerest form of flattery, offers further confirmation. By 1964 one other similar program had been developed. While no precise current figures are obtainable, we do know that the number of these programs has grown markedly. Last year's AMA listing ("Directory of Approved Internships and Residencies, 1968") indicates that there were 57 approved internship positions classified as "rotating–at least four months on psychiatry." A personal review of the corresponding individual hospital listings suggests that there are now four other institutions whose programs are at least roughly similar to ours, and which now accept at least two interns in that program, are teaching hospitals affiliated with medical schools, and also offer psychiatric residencies. In addition, there are at least four others meeting these latter criteria whose program comparability I am unable to judge.

What can we say about the future? For our own part, as I have by now made abundantly clear, we plan to continue our program until such time that external circumstances change. The recent jump in size was made on an experimental basis; and we may decide that we have overestimated the interest or that we cannot do full justice to this number of trainees. While we doubt that either will be the case, it will certainly be some years before we consider the possibility of a further enlargement, and I am inclined to think we are about at our maximum.

Similarly, I expect that both the number and size of other similar programs will continue to grow. Our success and that elsewhere would seem to make this inevitable. Other places will want to have these able young people in their programs, if only for a year. Unfortunately, I strongly suspect there is a paradox hidden in this competitive bandwagon. The particular applicant pool has been a special one. While it has shown some capacity to grow, I doubt seriously that it will ever become very large. As the number of similar programs increases one can predict that the applicants will become progressively more like the general pool of those seeking residencies. Certainly this will occur if this type of program becomes the modal one.

Competitiveness aside, I suspect that the forces operating broadly in medical education will relentlessly push our field in that direction. Certainly internships as currently designed will undergo further change. My own bet at the moment is that it will not be long before the internship disappears completely and is replaced by an additional year of residency. As I have explained, I feel that for psychiatry (and for a number of other specialties) this will be a mistake unless the first year of the residency includes several concentrated months of medicine. Yet I doubt that the trend can stop sharply at the midpoint represented by a program like ours. If only a segment of the top-flight centers offer a year of *straight* psychiatric training–be it called an internship or the first year of a four-year residency–the students will flock to these. The pressures of time and their eagerness to work in the specialty of their choice will be too difficult to resist. The issues which make the mixed program of value are too long-term, subtle and difficult for them to appreciate. The operation of the marketplace will force all of us to change. Thus my personal prediction is that programs of this type will not survive more than another 10-15 years–and this saddens me.

I cannot end on so depressing a note. For the present, we at Syracuse will continue to get much intellectual gratification and excitement from our program. And the future will bring plenty of alternatives in making adjustments in all our training programs to keep up with the pace of a changing world and a changing psychiatry. I hardly think that professors of psychiatry will ever want for challenge!

Note: Within the past few months, I have learned of three additional new mixed internship programs, meeting the criteria noted above, which will accept trainees for the forthcoming academic year. My prediction regarding the growth of such programs thus seems already borne out.

REFERENCES

1. Coggeshall, L. T. 1965. Planning for medical progress through education. Evanston, Illinois: The Association of American Medical Colleges.
2. Flexner, A. 1910. Medical education in the United States and Canada. Bulletin No. 4. New York: Carnegie Foundation for the Advancement of Teaching.

3. Grinker, R. R., Sr., et al. 1961. *The phenomena of depressions.* New York: Paul B. Hoeber, Inc.
4. Hollender, M. H. 1961. Psychiatry as part of a mixed internship. *JAMA,* 175 (February): 489.
5. ——, and Kaplan, E. A. 1965. Psychiatry as part of a mixed internship. *Arch. Gen. Psychiat.* 12:18.
6. Merton, R. K., et al. 1957. *The Student Physician,* Cambridge, Mass.: Harvard University Press.
7. Millis, J. S., et al. 1966. The Graduate Training of Physicians. Chicago: American Medical Association.

4. Teaching of Community Psychiatry in Psychiatric Residency Training Programs

Seymour R. Kaplan, M.D.

Any attempt to discuss teaching programs in community psychiatry is confronted with a lack of consensus about the parameters of the field even though the prevailing definitions of social psychiatry and community psychiatry can be more or less simply stated. Social psychiatry relates to the study of, and the theoretical formulations about, the social and environmental determinants of mental health and mental illness. Community psychiatry is the application of these studies and concepts to the development of programs for the prevention and treatment of mental illness. With some modifications I believe this definition reflects most of the existing opinions about the field of community psychiatry [7, 10, 17, 26, 29, 42, 49, 62, 63, 75, 83, 105]. The broadness of this definition is a result of the fact that the theories and practices in community psychiatry are still evolving, and little would be gained in attempting a more precise and specific definition. The issue of the parameters of community psychiatry will be approached instead by using either the references to the field which appear in the literature, or those based on my personal experiences with current practices. Also, I will briefly cover some of the historical and theoretical developments that have influenced the field of community psychiatry as well as the current circumstances within, and acting upon, medical institutions. It is important to consider these issues, even briefly, since any changes must be understood in terms of their relationship to preexisting programs and existing conditions if they are to be effectively integrated into existing programs. Resistance to change is inevitable, but if understood and seen in perspective, it can be resolved constructively.

PARAMETERS OF COMMUNITY PSYCHIATRY

In order to discuss appropriate training programs, the definition of community psychiatry needs to be supplemented by more practical guidelines. The references listed below are among those found in the literature or in current practices; they reflect what appear to be the viewpoints of the psychiatric community about social or community psychiatry rather than a consensus about the essential and defined parameters of these fields.

Frequent reference to the field has been based upon *therapeutic modalities* such as group and family therapy, therapeutic communities, or rehabilitation programs. There has been a trend to polarize training and treatment programs between those that focus on the dyadic situation and those that include all other treatment modalities, with the latter frequently associated with community psychiatric programs. There is nothing in the theory of social or community psychiatry to warrant placing these therapeutic modalities exclusively under this rubric, although the association has tended to emerge. Many psychiatric residency programs today do include training in the theory and practice of extradyadic therapeutic and paratherapeutic modalities. Their relevance to training in community psychiatry will be discussed below.

Another common reference to community psychiatry is in terms of the *organization of service delivery by geographic areas.* Service units are arranged so that patients from the same district, community, or neighborhood are treated at the same facility. This pattern is most common on the inpatient services of state hospitals that service widespread locales [45, 46, 77, 86, 99]. Selected wards are reserved for patients coming from a particular city or region of the state. At the other end of the service system, neighborhood outpatient units are being developed in some cities to provide services for patients within a small radius of a few blocks from the unit [53, 96].

The organization of service delivery by geographic areas had been implemented before the concept became mandated in federally sponsored community mental health centers, and there is nothing to warrant its exclusive application to this field. In defining community psychiatry, Linn [83] does use the "district aspect" as one of its essential features. The geographic arrangement of service delivery, however, is primarily a sensible administrative procedure for improving patient care.

Another frequently used basis for reference has reflected *governmental relationships to mental health institutions.* One of the major influences upon the developments in community psychiatry has come from federal planning and funding bodies, particularly the National Institute of Mental Health. The most notable example is the community mental health center concept [39, 45, 46, 95, 120]. Since the man who pays the piper often calls the tunes, the direction and guidelines for program developments established in Washington frequently have become the way of life in practice. Inevitably, no matter what the intent of the central planning bodies, these practices become institutionalized. Geographic delivery of services become "catchment areas" not always following a sensible pattern of patient flow; standard outpatient services are called after-care, and rehabilitation facilities and an alcove off an inpatient ward becomes a partial hospitalization service. If nothing else, it behooves us to understand the governmental procedures in order to intelligently appraise new programs.

However, I have not included this reference as a critique of the inevitable bureaucratic process of governmental machinery. I believe that the leadership taken by the federal planning groups was necessary and stems from the very complex problems of planning and finance in the entire medical care system. There are legitimate difficulties that prevent medical institutions from being responsive to the rapid changes in medical care and medical management that are required to maintain a high quality of medical practice. Medical centers, particularly the teaching institutions, are undergoing a reappraisal of their commitments in which the relationship to governmental bodies is a critical factor.

One of the more popular and common references to aspects of community psychiatry has related to *patterns of prevention* in the mental health-mental illness continuum of the individual—primary, secondary and tertiary [13, 15, 16, 18, 21, 31, 64]. Some programs, such as those which are referred to as secondary and tertiary prevention, are more or less traditional psychiatric programs. However, the major thrust of the programs in this category comes under what is referred to as primary prevention. This is a loosely defined concept which in its broadest application would include most of the significant aspects of the human environment within the parameters of mental health intervention. Indeed many of the innovative programs in community psychiatry have had their impetus from this concept [17, 22]. Its narrower application has been most clearly manifested in the role of the mental health consultant. This will be discussed below.

Still another reference to community psychiatry has been that of *concepts, planning, or programs for "defined populations."* This category is closely related to the preventive mental health approach and particularly to the traditions of public health [81]. The defined populations may be based upon categories of patients, i.e. addicts, geriatric patients, suicidal patients; or populations "at risk" because of developmental stress, i.e. preschool children, adolescents; or because of socioeconomic stress, i.e. the economically disadvantaged and minority groups [22, 28, 51, 57, 58, 61, 67, 69, 85, 87, 89, 117]. Program objectives and implementation often require the skills of epidemiologists and biostatisticians as well as clinical administrators knowledgeable about the formal and informal institutions with which the target populations are engaged. If psychiatric residents are to be trained for roles in this type of program, they must be sufficiently grounded in these areas in order to be able to utilize the skills of other professional disciplines.

References to community psychiatry may reflect *programs for training and utilization of mental health manpower.* In part this refers to programs for the training and utilization within the psychiatric setting of the related professional disciplines just mentioned, i.e. epidemiologists, biostatisticians, and mental health administrators. In addition I am referring to the training and utilization of nonprofessional staff in psychiatric programs [33, 54, 76, 79, 102, 103]. The utilization of nonprofessionals has been so markedly expanded, particularly in some community psychiatry programs in disadvantaged areas, that the nature of the program is strongly influenced by this staff [19, 52, 70, 82, 92]. One often cannot adequately evaluate these programs without knowledge of the skills and functions of the nonprofessional staff members.

The large scale development of this cadre of staff, not only in the psychiatric but in the other health and human services, is seen both as an important manpower resource and as a means of social and economic change [97, 101]. The federal government, which has been strongly supporting this development, has talked in terms of a million new career possibilities in the human services of which the health service is a large element. While the relevance of this development for psychiatric residency training is indirect, there are some specific aspects of the presence of a large number of nonprofessional staff that I will discuss below.

Although I have approached the above descriptions in the most general way, there are other concepts—planning or programs that are referred to under the social or community psychiatry rubric—which are not covered except under the broadest application of the preventive mental health or the public health reference. There is no overall categorization for these *new parameters;* for the most part they are experimental and tentative explorations. They are innovative either because program concepts from other disciplines have been newly applied or emphasized in the community psychiatry program, or because the innovative aspects may emanate from the psychiatric program itself. Among the innovative programs which appear to have the stamp of a mental health approach are those references to programs directed toward institutional change. One example would be the intervention in the educational system through the program initiated by Schiff and Kellam [113]. Another would be the community development objectives in the Lincoln Hospital Community Mental Health Center program [94, 95].

HISTORICAL DEVELOPMENT AND CURRENT ISSUES

The "moral treatment" that was practiced in a few mental hospitals around the year 1840 is often related to the background of the historical developments of community psychiatry. It was at that time that Dorothea Lynde Dix mounted an exposé of the squalid conditions that prevailed in most mental institutions. Despite these efforts mental hospitals during the 19th and early

20th century remained as large custodial institutions existing in deplorable circumstances. Adolf Meyer was one of the first to delineate some of the concepts of what we refer to today as community psychiatry. Meyer noted in 1913 that "the characteristic traits of a clinic for mental diseases should be first, service to the patient rather than to the administrative system; second, elaboration on the study of the diseases rather than the means of wholesale handling of patients; third, possibilities of following up the studies of nature's experiment beyond the hospital period, and preventive work through extramural effort outside the hospital" [45]. He also broached the issue of serving circumscribed units of population so that the social situations and dynamic factors that lead to mental illness could be explored for purposes of prevention.

Before World War II, there were indications of movements toward changes in mental institutions. These were manifested by the enlightened approach toward the severely mentally ill in England which resulted in the "open door" policies, by the work of a Dutchman, A. Querido, who developed a community-oriented program of home treatment, by large scale community-based programs for the mentally ill in the Soviet Union, and by other changes. However, it was not until after World War II that one could see evidence of major changes in the care of the mentally ill. The experiences of psychiatrists in the military services, some of which related to the developments in community psychiatry, have been noted by Daniels. He pointed out, "The beginnings of many principles currently utilized in community psychiatry are to be found in these military experiences; e.g., early recognition, treatment close to the source of the disability, crisis-oriented treatment promoting adaptation and return to duty and consultation to command about issues of general concern" [26]. The large number of individuals discharged from military services because of psychiatric disability, for which the country was unprepared, led to the marked expansion of Veterans Administration facilities. Because of superior facilities and staff, the Veterans Administration hospitals were able to provide improved patient care compared to the average state hospital. Furthermore, the Veterans Administration programs led to an increase in outpatient facilities and overall improvement of training of the various mental health professionals.

Another major development that had a marked impact on the trend in community psychiatry was the discovery and utilization of psychotropic drugs during the 1950s. With these drugs and the continuation of improved attitudes toward patient care, as in the development on a wide scale of such treatment approaches as the therapeutic community [66] and the use of partial hospitalization facilities [47, 123], there was a marked reduction of patients in mental institutions. Concomitant with this change in inpatient care there has been an increase in outpatient services since 1940. This increase, along with other expansions of mental health facilities and staff, was to a large measure the result of planning at the federal government level. In addition to funds for V.A. hospitals and facilities, the establishment of the National Institute of Mental Health led to grants and programs outside of hospitals and encouraged expansion of research and training projects. There has been a definite increase in the last twenty years of psychiatric residency training programs as well as involvement by the psychiatric faculty in medical school education.

In 1952, the community mental health concept in its present form was expressed by the Expert Committee on Mental Health of the World Health Organization. By 1961 the findings of the Joint Commission on Mental Illness and Health led to the publication of *Action For Mental Health* [65]. This resulted in 1963 in the enactment of Public Law 88-162–the "Mental Retardation Facilities and Community Mental Health Centers Construction Act of 1963." This formally launched the community mental health centers.

These recent developments in the field of psychiatry are paralleled by corresponding changes in the other health fields. The major goals of the community mental health center concept are the provisions for comprehensiveness and continuity of patient care and mental health services for all patients within a defined area who require it. These goals are directed to counteract the fragmentation of medical treatment which is prevalent to some extent in all the health services. This goal in the psychiatric field has been noted by the Joint Information Service: "It should be recognized that one of the stiffest challenges of the whole movement [the community mental health center] is the need for many agencies to coordinate now separate programs; this will require a magnitude of compromise and cooperation that staggers the imagination" [46]. There have been changes recently in other health services with objectives similar to those in the mental health field. As Bandler has stated, "In recent years the medical schools and the Association of American Medical Colleges have been reexamining their goals in the light of the increase of knowledge and of society's needs for health care. One result has been the acceptance by a number of medical schools of responsibility for comprehensive health care for a limited geographic area of the community. The Association of American Medical Colleges and the medical schools have been vigorous in the recognition and response to social issues and in their relationship to the public bodies whose decisions and policies impinge so critically on medical education" [5].

The issue of social and community commitment by universities is of course very much in the forefront of current developments in the educational sphere. Educational institutions themselves are being pressed by faculty and students for changes in administration and curriculum. The marked increase of students participating in political and educational affairs, in part stimulated by the Vietnam war, has affected the universities in general.

Prior to and since World War II there has been increasing attention to social legislation, which has recently been focused on programs for disadvantaged populations. Among the programs that have direct bearing on community psychiatry are those sponsored by the Office of Economic Opportunity, notably the neighborhood service centers and neighborhood health centers, which have sometimes been under the direction of university medical centers [53, 121]. These programs are attempting to develop improved health service delivery to low income and minority groups. The concern with improvement of services has included all the human services provided by governmental agencies. One of the recent important developments along this line has been the Model Cities program which attempts to deal with the fragmentation of all the human services [96]. On an administrative level this attempt to consolidate and integrate the diverse bureaucratic procedures and agencies involved in the human services, particularly those in disadvantaged communities, is probably one of the most important and challenging issues of today. The importance of these changes for providing expanded and more effective health, educational, labor, housing, and welfare programs is made more urgent by the increasing unrest over civil rights issues.

The present administration in Washington has expressed the intent to expand the Model Cities program. Since future funding for community mental health centers is likely to tie in with the development of these programs, the impact of the civil rights movement upon community psychiatry programs will become more evident. Among the issues that require urgent attention in these programs are methods of relating to community developments so that programs can be appropriately responsive to these developments. This necessitates a variety of skills in administration, business practices and fiscal management, public relations, and program planning beyond the competence of even the most sophisticated medical departments, or for that matter, most medical centers. But beyond professional skills there appears to be a need for new institutional structures that can not only encompass such diverse professional skills, but also function within, or outside of, entrenched bureaucracies, both public and private. This will probably take the form of an intra or interuniversity corporate structure formed in collaboration with community lay boards that will draw upon the resources of many interrelated disciplines.

Just how a medical department and its teaching programs will relate to this development is still in the early talking stage. However, the need for a reshaping of university departments both on the undergraduate and graduate level had been recognized long before the current pressures for change were being brought by the public and private community. The growth and development of the theories and practices in the behavioral and physical sciences has proliferated at such a rapid pace that frequently the existing teaching structures no longer have any meaning. We are now undergoing a major realignment of disciplines into more functional and organic entities.

Lastly, with regard to other issues impinging upon current health and mental health practices, it might be additionally noted that the stage for changes in medical practices responsive to the public and private need was set many years ago with the creation of health protection measures. Closely tied in with the labor movements of the 1930s, but also stimulated by government and private insurance plans, the role of third party carriers in payment of medical costs has been rapidly expanding. With inevitable increases in medicaid legislation and improved fringe benefit plans, the payment through third party carriers will be the major method of payment for health and mental health services in the near future. This could mean that the consumer response to medical practices may play a major role in shaping these practices which will act as an effective leveling influence over class, racial or ethnic considerations. By distinguishing the consumer of services from the provider of services, it can clarify some of the current confusions about the community's role in establishing patterns of health services delivery.

THEORETICAL CONSIDERATIONS

The following are some major developments that I believe have had bearing on current practices in community psychiatry. The influence of psychopharmacology and humanistic approaches upon the treatment and care of the severely mentally ill has been noted. Within the area of psychoanalytic ego psychology, the work of Hartman [55] on adaptation and "conflict-free" spheres of ego-functioning, and the work of Erikson [34] on the epigenetic aspects of psychosocial adaptation are among many notable contributions. Their work, and those of other psychoanalytic theorists, have continued Freud's original concepts about the structural aspects of ego development and the relationship between individual ego functioning and the organization of significant social groups.

Relevant contributions to current practices in community psychiatry have come from clinicians who have utilized group and family therapy. Their clinical work in small group process, supplemented by that of behavioral scientists in social systems theory, has had a significant impact. Another major element has been derived from child psychiatry but since community psychiatry programs and child psychiatry programs are often combined, this paper will not be further addressed to the contributions of child psychiatry. However, it should be noted that the studies in child development and developmental theory in general are among the most promising areas from which the new parameters in community psychiatry may hope to gain definition and clarity.

GENERAL TRAINING ISSUES

At a time when residency training programs are overscheduled with a diversity of subjects and training objectives, one might wonder whether this is a propitious time to discuss additions to the curriculum. However, this is a time of institutional change particularly in the educational areas, and it appears that there is little choice but to respond. The initiative will probably come from curriculum changes at the medical school level which will affect psychiatric residency programs as much, if not more, than other specialities. Current change in the Albert Einstein College of Medicine curriculum relevant to psychiatric residency training is reflected in proposed additions in the behavioral sciences and in the early development of tracks for students interested in specialized medical disciplines. With such change, residents in psychiatry will enter their training at a much more advanced level of experience than they do currently. This will significantly affect the residency curriculum and should allow for a more sensible scheduling of programs. Therefore, I look upon any immediate alterations in residency training as an interim measure pending the outcome of changes in the medical school programs.

Some of the prevailing problem issues will remain regardless of these changes. One notable dilemma is the conflict that arises over service commitments and teaching commitments. This is particularly pertinent to the field of community psychiatry since one influence on its development directly relates to the efforts of governmental planning bodies to induce university teaching centers to increase their service commitments. The need for the expansion is obvious, but the question of methods of implementation is complex. One issue is clear, however—that recruitment and training of staff for expanded programs is a crucial problem, and that expansion at the expense of training would be extremely short-sighted. The failure of the governmental funding bodies to provide adequate funds for teaching is one of the major errors that must be corrected if their well-intended plans are to have any chance to develop. The failure to make adequate provision for research and evaluation is equally crucial.

There are other subjects being explored in general residency training that are relevant to all aspects of training, e.g. the examination of pedagogical techniques currently used in the medical field. This includes a critical appraisal of the didactic methods of seminars and lectures, the possible role of programmed teaching, and the potential uses of videotape and other teaching techniques. The area of the learning situation itself is being influenced by group process techniques, notably the sensitivity or "T" group exercises [3, 14, 40, 68, 118]. The impact of the more active participation of students in policies and practices of educational institutions is being felt in medical education as well. These issues, I feel, have as much bearing upon teaching programs as the content of the curriculum. Lastly, I'd like to stress with regard to *any* program, particularly any modification of existing programs or the introduction of new programs, that it is the commitment and interest of the faculty that will determine its effectiveness as much as any reordering of the content or method of teaching.

TRAINING PROGRAMS FOR COMMUNITY PSYCHIATRY

For purposes of exposition the educational areas for community psychiatry will be discussed in terms of three roles: the clinical practitioner, the mental health consultant, and the administrator—a general category of roles which include administration, program planning and community development. The training for the role of clinical practitioner in community psychiatry does not deviate from existing training practices but emphasizes aspects of current training. The training for the role of mental health consultant and the administrative roles in program planning, community development or other specialized aspects of the mental health field does represent a departure from most existing residency training programs. In discussing specific training programs for these roles, I will limit myself to the programs occurring during the three year general residency period [8, 9, 10, 23, 24, 25, 27, 30, 35, 37, 48, 49, 50, 51, 56, 60, 62, 63, 73, 74, 75, 90, 100, 105, 107, 112, 114, 116].

Training for the Role of the Clinical Practitioner

In most existing training programs there are clinical assignments which are as necessary for a background in community psychiatry as in any of the other clinical specialties of psychiatry. The assignment to individual, intensive, long-term therapy is a core training experience whatever the resident's ultimate career objectives. However, this section will be limited to a discussion of clinical assignments to the care of the acutely ill patient, to therapeutic work with the patient in relation to his significant environment, and to assignments to the follow-up care of the chronically ill patient.

In the care of the acutely ill patient who is seen in the emergency service, the resident in the Lincoln program is assigned to the *patient* rather than to the *service.* The purpose is to provide the resident with continuous patient contact through the acute and subacute treatment of the patient's illness regardless of the service in which the treatment is offered. This may include an overnight acute service for those patients requiring two or three days of inpatient care, partial hospitalization service, or a referral to the outpatient services. On the average, the resident follows the patient assigned to him for about four weeks, which is sufficient time to observe some reconstitution from acute illness of most patients selected for this short-term contract. At the end of the four weeks the patient is transferred to staff members. This training assignment, along with the experiences on the inpatient services during the first year, each of which is for six months, provides the resident with continuous contact with severely ill patients during the acute and subacute phases and during the long-term reconstitution from illness.

On the inpatient and the partial hospitalization service (which is the major transitional treatment resource for the acutely ill patient not requiring extended inpatient care), the resident participates in a variety of extradyadic therapeutic settings [93]. In addition to direct clinical treatment in formal small group therapy or family therapy, patients are involved in therapeutic community meetings and paratherapeutic group activities. For the most part during the first year the residents do not conduct group therapy or therapeutic community meetings, but act as observers or participants as indicated. Residents who are assigned to work with families are supervised in this experience. They also participate in multidisciplinary staff meetings concerning the patient's behavior in dyadic and extradyadic settings.

During the second year of both the Jacobi and the Lincoln-Einstein programs, residents are assigned to the follow-up care of patients who come to the clinic as a referral by other medical departments, through the emergency room, or from the inpatient services. Most of these patients are chronically ill, many have been hospitalized, and most are receiving medication. In a majority of clinics required to serve this patient population, patients are seen briefly at monthly intervals or longer primarily for purposes of having prescriptions for medication renewed. Some years ago at Jacobi and subsequently at Lincoln, patients requiring long-term follow-up care were referred to a therapeutic group program. The group approaches utilized in this program have varied from discussion groups, which are similar to formal therapy groups, to groups in which social or work activities are the major therapeutic modality, either separately or combined with discussion periods [76, 115]. The programs have been administered and conducted by nonmedical staff, primarily social workers or psychologists. There is extensive utilization of nonprofessional staff who are trained by the Einstein Department of

Psychiatry as adjunct group leaders. In the Jacobi program the nonprofessional staff are recruited from among white middle-class women [79] and at the Lincoln program the nonprofessional staff are black and Puerto Rican men and women recruited from the lower economic level [82].

During the first year, whether in reference to the acute, subacute or chronic phase of illness, it is recommended that the teaching include two aspects of the ego process inherent in the restitution from severe illness: the nature of the individual ego process in the dyadic situation, and the social or group process during restitution. In both instances attention is directed to the structure and process of ego functioning as well as the dynamic, "conflict" aspect. The role of individual ego functioning during restitution from psychosis is familiar, although often not sufficiently stressed. While any dichotomy of ego process between dyadic and group process is artificial, and specific theories to bridge the two processes are lacking, one can provide a practical training experience based on observations that relate in some measure to one or the other of the phenomena.

The relevance of this combined emphasis on dyadic and group developmental process is that the resident can be introduced to the nature of behavior in small groups, composed of patients and therapist, patients and general staff, and staff alone. The differences in leadership, attitudes toward authority and peers, and methods of achieving the different goals can be compared to the similarity of process and structure in various group settings. Sufficient knowledge of the differences and similarities in identifications and object relationships, and the nature of transference and countertransference between the dyadic and the group setting can provide a groundwork for future competence in these areas [1, 2, 11, 36, 41, 68, 71, 72, 98, 108, 109, 110]. Work with family group therapy supplements the study of small group dynamics and process. In addition, the resident's own experience in a sensitivity or "T" group can have value in rounding out these experiences, provided the focus is on educational, not therapeutic, goals [68, 122].

In summary, the first year training, with minor modifications of existing programs and teaching emphasis, can provide an important background for the role of clinical practitioner in community psychiatry. By making the assignments to the emergency services a vital and significant part of the teaching program, the concept of continuity of care can be related to the ego processes in the recovery from illness and demonstrated by clinical experiences. By including assignments to extradyadic settings and emphasizing relevant theory, the resident's appreciation of environmental determinants in illness and recovery from illness can be firmly anchored in clinical experiences.

During the second year, in assignments to the care of the chronically ill patient, the resident has direct contact with a variety of rehabilitative programs needed for this patient population [12]. Since group treatment programs of this type play an important part in the development of services for community mental health centers [78] they fill a gap in the usual residency training assignments. Furthermore, the resident's work with other disciplines, with which he became familiar in the first year, is expanded. In the Lincoln program, vocational training experiences in presheltered workshops, as well as considerable attention to the expediting of problems around welfare, housing, etc., provide the resident with exposure to the complex of service needs of multiproblemed families [6, 119]. The resident is able to compare his earlier group experiences, which were focused more specifically upon direct therapeutic measures, with the use of group settings in which educational and socialization techniques are used. At the same time, the basic similarities of small group processes in all settings can be observed, despite the differences in leadership, authority relationships, and goals of treatment.

The resident-supervisor relationship remains the most effective teaching method in clinical psychiatry whatever the specialty [32, 38]. (The supervisory relationship will be discussed in greater detail in the section on the role of mental health consultant.) I think it imperative that this teaching method be maintained, even at the expense of seminars and conferences. The supervision of several residents in a group has some advantages that can supplement individual supervision. It has been observed that the supervisor who has time to become familiar with the therapeutic milieu in which the resident works can be most helpful in offering additional insights concerning the interrelationship of individual and social determinants [25]. Since I believe that a thorough background in small group theory is an important complement to training in individual psychoanalytic theory, supervisors knowledgeable in both fields would help avoid an unnecessary dichotomy of the fundamentals of the unconscious and preconscious determinants of pathology and its relationship to transference phenomena. This will accrue benefits in training for the resident whether his career objective is private or community practice.

The previous programs and teaching assignments fall within existing models of residency training. Assignments to the programs discussed below are given during the third year and are electives for interested residents. In most instances, these programs deviate from the medical model in that the approach does not focus upon the patient-doctor relationship or necessarily set the individual patient (or client) in the central role of the services rendered. For purposes of exposition, I will discuss these programs and their teaching assignments first in terms of the psychiatrist as a mental health consultant and then in terms of the issue of authority and power in programs, concepts, or planning that reflect other new parameters of community psychiatry besides the role of the mental health consultant.

As a background for the discussion of these programs, the reader may wish to review the summary of the teaching programs in community psychiatry of sixteen training centers in the GAP report, *Education for Community Psychiatry* [42]. That summary indicates the prominent part that public health programs play in training in community psychiatry [4, 9, 20, 80, 84, 91, 106].

The Psychiatrist as a Mental Health Consultant

I would distinguish this role from the role of the psychiatrist as a specialist who confers on a specific individual's clinical problems. The role of the psychiatrist as a mental health consultant may, and often does, include direct consultation and services for patients or client referrals from the consultee agency. However, as the concept is now evolving [15], the mental health consultant sees his functions as extending beyond such direct services. They now include educational goals, as, for example, in educating the consultee about the mental health aspects of referred patients or clients. They also include attempts by the mental health consultant to influence the patterns of services of the consultee agency along programmatic lines. For example, he may induce the agency to consider preventive mental health objectives, or to undertake direct therapeutic measures within its program. In these latter instances, he is functioning as a program consultant. Often this occurs by direct request, at times, indirectly.

Educational goals and programmatic goals call for different methods and commitments. There are differences of methods and commitments in mental health consultation for the psychiatrist who advises and assists a school principal on programs for the early detection of and approach to children suffering from a school phobia, and for the psychiatrist who helps in planning for special programs for young adolescents with a director of a group service agency, such as a settlement house [111]. But most of all I would like to comment on the differences from the traditional training situation for the resident who is learning about these methods and commitments when his supervisor is *not* a member of the faculty of his training center. I believe that consideration of training methods or the training situation is more pertinent than the curriculum content at this time.

It has been observed that the role of the mental health consultant deviates from the medical model. It also tends to be the case that the teaching methods currently used in general residency programs for this role deviate from the traditional methods in medical internships and residency training. This is so primarily because training for the role of mental health consultant is based upon the methods used by public health and social work schools. The major training in clinical psychiatry is the supervision the resident receives from the teacher of the diagnostic and treatment methods, which he then applies to patients to whom he has been assigned and for whom he assumes responsibility. The same type of supervision cannot be used in the nonclinical situation such as that of the mental health consultant. Except for unusual circumstances, a resident cannot be assigned responsibilities for program consultation as described above in the same manner as he is assigned to the treatment of patients in clinical psychiatry. There is an inherent difference in the contractual relationship between the doctor and a patient, and the consultant and consultee.

However, there is another difference between the clinical teaching situation of the school of medicine and the schools of public health and social work which is partly inherent to the subject areas and partly a matter of the role of these training institutions and their relationship to service commitments. The school of medicine, no matter how circumscribed in its service commitments, has members of its faculty directly responsible for the clinical services within which the clinical teaching is provided, and usually has administrative responsibility as well. The schools of public health and of social work to a large extent depend for their training assignments upon the use of field placements for which their faculty has no administrative and usually no professional responsibility. They have developed, however, highly structured and sophisticated relationships between their faculties and the administrative and professional staff of the services to which their students are assigned. In recent years, as psychiatric residency training centers have undertaken to teach in the nonclinical areas, they have also used field placements, but often without any defined relationship between psychiatric faculty and professional staff of the services to which the residents are assigned. Furthermore, where the teaching goal is similar to a training program in a public health or social work curriculum which assigns a student full time for a year or at least for nine months to a field placement, the psychiatric resident is often assigned to an agency, school or court on a half-day basis for three to six months or less [42]. As a consequence, the training for the role of mental health consultant in a psychiatric residency program often does not have one of the best qualities of medical school teaching—a faculty member and institution which have responsibility for the services *within* which the resident learns. Nor does it have one of the best qualities of the public health or social work school—a faculty who are sophisticated in negotiating a training situation for their students *outside* their institution. I am making this point about the nature of the training situation because of the importance of the teaching supervisor as a model of identification for the resident. As Rosenbaum has noted [104], the resident's concern about his professional identity is a prime issue that must be considered in any training program. The student-supervisor relationship, particularly in intensive, individual, long-term therapy, has been one of the most consistently positive learning and growth experiences for residents that I have observed through many years of contact with residency training programs. The supervisor usually has a central role on the teaching faculty. However, at the present time the supervisor of residents at a field placement is usually not a faculty member, or he has been given a token appointment and is not meaningfully related to the teaching program. There are, of course, very practical issues about the relevant qualifications and skills of the supervisors in the field placement agencies in terms of the standards of a psychiatric department of a medical school. But I think that the impact of the situation in terms of the resident's concern about his identity must be considered in teaching and planning for the role of mental health consultant, lest a great deal of effort be wasted in overlooking this fundamental issue of the learning situation.

In summary, I would like to suggest the following. If the teaching goal for the role of mental health consultant is *to educate* the psychiatric resident about the nature of the operations of the formal or the informal agencies and institutions in the community, I can see the value of brief unaffiliated assignments in the field. If the goal is to teach the resident *how to educate* the staff of the consultee agency, or to help in program development, then I think residency programs must meet two conditions. They must first recognize how sophisticated even the more limited objective of education of a consultee agency is, to say nothing of the role of program consultant, and allow sufficient time for training in the principles of these roles. One assignment is preferable to a number of rotations, since there are basic principles of mental health consultation which apply generally. Second, they should have or develop a consultation service in which their teaching faculty has a significant commitment to an agency or agencies. I believe that the faculty of the program within which the resident is learning should have a defined obligation to provide a consultation service that, while not the same as a clinical commitment, has a comparable quality of responsibility. An alternative is to negotiate joint faculty positions at a high academic level for the supervisory and teaching staff at both the medical school and the participating agencies.

In addition to the importance of the faculty as models of identification, there is another reason for a teaching institution to assume responsibility for providing services, even if in a circumscribed manner. In many applied scientific fields today, the gap between theory and practice is often considerable. This is certainly true for the psychiatric field. Unless the faculty of a teaching institution is meaningfully involved in the practices for which it is training students, there is an inevitable tendency for the curriculum to become isolated from the significant clinical developments in their respective areas. In the past, this was avoided in the medical schools by the prominent place on the faculty of the clinician-teacher. With the changes in recent years that have seen the clinician-teacher lose his prominence, the gap between theory and practice has become so marked that it is, I think, one of the major contributory factors to the current crisis in medical education. I do not think that the concern for maintaining basic research and for protecting appropriate faculty from being overburdened by service responsibilities should obscure the issue of the consequences of medical institutions which do not give adequate attention to the application of theory to clinical and nonclinical practice.

The Issue of Authority and Power

The role of the psychiatrist in community psychiatry beyond the role of the clinical practitioner encompasses such functions as administration, program planning, community development, and so on. In this section about the new parameters in community psychiatry I would like to attempt to consider some basic common issues related to the change in functions from the traditional medical model. Rosenbaum and Zwerling remark that "once the focus of attention shifts from the patient as an individual to the patient as a member of a group, the psychiatrist no longer has the same feelings of professional security and superiority with his nonmedical colleagues as does his more traditionally oriented counterpart" [105].

There are many issues involved in this shift of functions for the psychiatrist that need extensive discussion, not the least of which is whether the shift to new parameters is appropriate to begin with. However, proceeding on the assumption that some change is inevitable, I will take a leaf from a recent GAP report. In discussing the role of the psychiatrist when he functions outside of defined areas, the GAP report, *The Dimensions of Community Psychiatry* concludes, "negotiations may be the key concept in this role. The psychiatrist-participant negotiates with others as his peers about spheres of influence and the sharing of authority and responsibility. For example, the chairman of a department of psychiatry negotiates with his colleagues for curriculum teaching time. Conflicts of interest are settled by mediation or by arbitration" [43]. I am inclined to agree with the report although I would here like to stress the issue of authority and power in teaching programs since I believe it to be the issue that is fundamental to any negotiations. The understanding of the role of power in the human situation has been generally neglected in residency training and in the theory and practice of psychiatry. It was Freud's difficulty in "negotiating" with his gifted friend and follower, Alfred Adler, that in part resulted in the omission from the main body of psychoanalytic theory of Adler's views about the basic role of power in the dynamics of human behavior. Caplan makes some rather pointed observations on "the methods of achieving and manipulating power and influence in public life in order to modify the conduct of affairs" [16]. He is rather cryptic about the limitations of psychiatrists in this area. It may very well be that in the final analysis the art of negotiation and manipulation of power is a matter of life-long experience that cannot be taught. However, there is, I believe, a degree of ineptitude in these areas among the health professionals, from which the psychiatrist is not exempt, and which may be to some extent a by-product of our training situation.

Some years ago it came to my attention that the reaction of psychiatric residents to the learning situation would often be manifested by an ambivalent reaction to the authority of the teaching faculty. This appears to be a normative response to anxiety about the learning situation and probably no different basically than that of other students. It is intensified by the unique responsibilities of residents in the hospital service system and, as Zinberg and Friedman [122] have speculated, probably heightened by the nature of the subject matter that the psychiatric resident is learning. As I have commented above, the teacher plays a vital role as a model of identification for the resident and it is understandable that ambivalent feelings toward the faculty become activated under these stressful circumstances. Idealization and denigration reactions toward the faculty are readily observable among residents, particularly during their first two years, and these reactions may interfere with the acquisition of knowledge and the development of skills. Holt makes a similar observation about psychiatric residents during the training period [59]. In an earlier paper I described how a modified sensitivity or "T" group can be utilized in a residency training program to demonstrate the ambivalent reactions to the authority of the teacher [68]. This teaching method may also serve as a means of learning about the distinctions between normative and pathological adaptation toward authority in institutional settings. This is a distinction that can best be demonstrated in the extradyadic setting and is a crucial concept with which the clinical practitioner in community psychiatry must be thoroughly familiar.

However, recent developments in the climate of educational institutions make it clear that any modification of teaching methods such as the one described above will not suffice to help clarify ambivalent reactions of residents to the teaching faculty when the training situation involves roles beyond that of the clinician. I will give a specific example of this below. In general, I am referring to training programs in which conflicts arise over the issue of the authority and power of the medical institution itself. Any ambivalent reactions projected upon the teacher, or about the issue, are too readily rationalized by the political aspects of the situation. In the previously mentioned paper I had observed the tendency to use a political metaphor as a symbolic expression of ambivalent reactions to the learning situation: "In the early meetings, the residents, despite some bickering, had tended to interact as a unit, but in recent meetings, dissension had split the members into conflicting subgroups, apparently around the pros and cons of the training method. . . . The arguments between the contending subgroups had more of the tone of a political convention or a dispute over ideological beliefs than a scientific appraisal of professional technique" [68]. At that time the politicalization of the training situation served as a symbolic expression which most of the residents could identify and contrast to the reality of the learning situation. It was a more readily identifiable metaphor than the more primitive symbolic representations of early object relationships that were also manifested. Since the learning situation in which this occurred was a clinical training program in group therapy, the inappropriateness of a political reaction to the learning situation was readily demonstrated. Such was not the case in the events that occurred recently at the Lincoln Hospital Mental Health Services. I will describe these briefly to illustrate the problem of residency training in programs that fall outside of the traditional role models.

The events at the Lincoln Hospital Mental Health Services grew out of two important innovations in the program: the training and utilization of a large number of nonprofessional staff [70], and movements in the area of community development which culminated in the agreement by the National Institute of Mental Health and the Community Mental Health Board of New York City to fund directly the Hunts Point Multi-Service Center to provide outpatient mental health services in its area. The Hunts Point Multi-Service Center is a community corporation in the South Bronx in one of the Model Cities areas of New York City. The corporation was initiated and developed entirely by elected representatives of the area. The funds allocated to the corporation are part of the funds for a community mental health center staffing grant which had been awarded to the Lincoln Hospital Mental Health Services. The arrangement to have a community corporation directly funded and in control of the mental health outpatient services for its area was done with the active collaboration of the Lincoln program. It is, to my knowledge, the first arrangement of its kind in this country in which a community-elected corporation directly controls a mental health service component of a community mental health center in collaboration with a university medical school. Despite this development, or perhaps partly because of it, some members of the Lincoln Mental Health staff staged a sit-in protesting the failure to achieve a greater degree of community participation and/or control. The issues leading to this reaction include problems stemming from the awesome bureaucratic red tape of the New York City municipal hospital system, complicated even further by the new and changing federal guidelines for a community mental health center; the problems of personnel and labor-management practices in a university that had just signed a union contract; and outgrowths of local political issues in a disadvantaged community torn by civil rights conflicts, in which the unresolved issue of community control in the educational system had left a bitter residue. The point I wish to illustrate is that whatever the merits of the protest, a few staff members with personal, political goals unrelated to the specific program issues of the Lincoln Hospital Mental Health Service were able to involve many other staff members in their strategy. While the majority of staff involved in the protest were nonprofessionals, a number of professionals, including psychiatric residents, participated in the protest for a time, with the result that there was a temporary suspension of the services and a serious setback in the program.

The residents, as well as some of the other staff who became involved, were unusually naive about local political issues and made little effort to be informed about them or to distinguish them from those issues specific to conflicts among the staff. For example, the distinction between community control and staff control of programs and policies was obscured. Many of the staff members, whether involved in the protest or not, favored an increased voice by the community in program policies; this had in fact been the stated objective of the program. Those who were involved in the protest were under the impression that the issue of community control was the primary agenda for all the dissident staff. However, the strategy of some of the leaders of the protest was to establish staff control and there occurred in effect a maneuver by a small self-selected staff group to take over the authority of the program and to establish a power base for themselves. This specific issue of an internal staff conflict over power was obscured by the emotionality of the general issue of community control. The protest rapidly escalated beyond the staff and became a political conflict involving many groups outside the community. Suffice to say that a rather complicated situation existed which even a sophisticated participant would have been hard put to understand. However most of the participants made little effort on their own to obtain the facts, and it is this lack of attention to, and interest in, the specifics to which I am addressing myself.

Whatever their political convictions, it was not the intent of the psychiatric residents to subvert the teaching program or the capacity of their teachers to supervise their work. Nevertheless, this is what occurred to the detriment of all involved. Part of the explanation of the residents' behavior can be described as a result of their overidentification with the nonprofessional staff and the polarization of their ambivalent reactions into a good-bad object relationship projected upon the "establishment," personified by senior members of the faculty. I should make it clear that the residents who became involved are among the more highly regarded in the training program and who, in their supervised work, had not shown any propensity to these defense mechanisms in intensive long-term individual therapy or other therapeutic situations. However, because of their use of denial and rationalization and because of the reality of the political developments, it was not possible to discuss the issues with the residents objectively, or to turn their reactions to the advantage of the learning process.

Whatever else can be said about these events at Lincoln, it is clear that the training situation could not productively encompass these developments, and that more thought about the assignments of residents to programs of this nature is necessary.

I would like to make clearer what the training aspects are with which I am concerned. I am not referring to the issue of radical political activism of students. While I am concerned about the potentially destructive effects of such actions upon a resident or a program, such actions are a matter of the individual resident's prerogatives, and he must answer for them to his own conscience or to the authorities, if extreme actions occasion that. Nor am I referring to the question of the actual role of authority on the part of a teacher who has administrative responsibility. What I am referring to is how, and by what means, a training program can help develop the kind of sophistication about issues of authority and power that many of the programs in community psychiatry require. It is clear in the events that developed at Lincoln, in similar events with which I am familiar, and in other less dramatic circumstances that the residents often do not adequately clarify for themselves whether their actions are as citizens or as professionals, nor do they appear to be adequately aware of the implications and consequences of their actions for themselves and others. In the instance of resident applicants whom I have interviewed who were dropped from other training programs or were pressured to leave other programs, it was all too clear that they were unprepared for that eventuality. In some, the problem was the individual resident who would have had difficulty apart from his social actions. In others, this did not appear to be the case. I do not know whether I am addressing myself to unrealistic expectations for a residency training program, or for the senior professional for that matter, when it is still not clear what the area of competence is to which the training is directed. The GAP report notes, "It is apparent that the psychiatrist can participate and collaborate with others as a psychiatrist (rather than as a citizen, for example) only if his competence in his field is recognized and he acts within that area of competence." But the report goes on to add, "In collaborative situations—and this may be particularly relevant in poverty programs—the psychiatrist will have to define his area of competence as he goes along" [43].

REFERENCES

1. Appelbaum, S. 1963. The pleasure and reality principles in group process teaching. *British Journal of Medical Psychology,* vol. 36.
2. Arlow, J. 1961. Ego psychology and the study of mythology. *Journal of the American Psychoanalytic Association,* vol. 9.
3. Astrachan, B., and Redlich, F. Leadership ambiguity and its effect on residents' "study group." *International Journal of Group Psychotherapy,* in press.
4. Baler, L. 1965. Community mental health: training program in a school of public health. *Community Mental Health Journal,* vol. 1, no. 3 (Fall).
5. Bandler, B. 1968. The American Psychoanalytic Association and community psychiatry. *American Journal of Psychiatry,* vol. 124 (February).
6. Bauman, G., and Douthit, V. 1968. Vocational rehabilitation and community mental health in deprived urban areas. *Journal of Rehabilitation* (Nov.-Dec.).
7. Bellak, L. 1964. Community psychiatry: the third psychiatric revolution, in Bellak, L. ed., *Handbook of community psychiatry and community mental health.* New York: Grune and Stratton, Inc.
8. Berlin, I. 1965. Training in community psychiatry: its relation to clinical psychiatry. *Community Mental Health Journal,* vol. 1, no. 4 (Winter).
9. Bernard, V. 1960. A training program in community psychiatry: integrating trends in public health and administration. *Mental Hospital,* vol. 11 (May).
10. ——. 1964. Education for community psychiatry in a university medical center (with emphasis on the rationale and objectives of training), in Bellak, L. ed., *Handbook of community psychiatry and community mental health.* New York: Grune and Stratton, Inc.
11. Bion, W. 1959. *Experiences in groups.* New York: Basic Books.
12. Black, B. and Benney, C. 1969. *Rehabilitation: the schizophrenic syndrome.* New York: Grune and Stratton.
13. Bower, E. 1963. Primary prevention of mental and emotional disorders. *American Journal of Orthopsychiatry,* vol. 33.
14. Bradford, L., Gibb, J. and Benne, K. 1964. *T-Group theory and laboratory method.* New York: Wiley and Sons.
15. Caplan, G. 1959. Concepts of mental health and consultation. Washington, D.C.: U.S. Children's Bureau, no. 373.
16. ——. 1961. *Prevention of mental disorders in children.* New York: Basic Books.

17. _____. 1961. *An approach to community mental health.* New York: Grune and Stratton.
18. _____. 1964. *Principles of preventive psychiatry.* New York: Basic Books.
19. Christmas, J. J. 1966. Group methods in training and practice: nonprofessional mental health personnel in a deprived community. *American Journal of Orthopsychiatry,* vol. 36, no. 3.
20. Coleman, J. V., et al. 1965. A teaching program in public health psychiatry. *American Journal of Psychiatry,* vol. 122 (September).
21. Community psychology. 1966. Boston Conference on the Education of Psychologists for Community Mental Health, Boston, Massachusetts.
22. Cowen, E., Gardner, E., and Zax, M. 1967. *Emergent approaches to mental health problems.* New York: Meredith Publishing Co.
23. Daniels, R. S. 1962. Current trends in psychiatric medical education. *Chicago Medicine,* vol. 65 (August).
24. _____. 1963. Education and training within and without the hospital. *Hospital Program* vol. 43 (September).
25. _____. 1965. The integration of community psychiatry training in a traditional psychiatric residency. *Mental Hygiene,* vol. 49 (January).
26. _____. 1966. Community psychiatry—a new profession, a developing subspecialty, or effective clinical psychiatry. *Community Mental Health Journal,* vol. 2, no. 1.
27. Davis, D., et al. 1968. Introducing the community to medical students and residents: an evaluation of a field trip program. *Journal of Medical Education,* vol. 43 (January).
28. Duhl, L. 1967. What mental health services are needed for the poor? In *Poverty and mental health,* ed. Greenblatt, Emery and Glueck. Psychiatric Research Reports of the American Psychiatric Association (January).
29. Dunham, H. 1965. Community psychiatry. *Archives of general psychiatry,* vol. 12.
30. Ehrenthal, O. F. 1967. A critique of psychiatric training programs: historical perspective and future trends. *International Journal of Neuropsychiatry,* vol. 3 (April).
31. Eisenberg, L., and Gruenberg, E. 1961. The current status of secondary prevention in child psychiatry. *American Journal of Orthopsychiatry,* vol. 31.
32. Ekstein, R., and Wallerstein, R. 1958. *The teaching and learning of psychotherapy.* New York: Basic Books.
33. Ellsworth, R. 1968. *Non-professionals in psychiatric rehabilitation.* New York: Meredith Publishing Company.
34. Erickson, E. 1959. Identity and the life cycle. *Psychological Issues,* vol. 1, monograph 1.
35. Errera, P., et al. 1967. The training of residents in a community psychiatric clinic. *Mental Hygiene,* vol. 51 (April).
36. Ezriel, H. 1950. A psychoanalytic approach to group treatment. *British Journal of Medical Psychology,* vol. 23.
37. Felix, R. H. 1966. The preparation of a community-oriented psy-

chiatrist. *American Journal of Psychiatry,* vol. 122, supplement 2-7 (June).
38. Fleming, J., and Benedek, T. 1964. Supervision: a method of teaching psychoanalysis. *Psychoanalytic Quarterly,* vol. 33.
39. Foley, A., and Sanders, D. 1966. Theoretical considerations for the development of the community mental health center concept. *American Journal of Psychiatry,* vol. 122, no. 9 (March).
40. Frank, J. 1964. Training Groups and therapy groups. In *T-Group theory and laboratory method,* ed. Bradford, L. New York: John Wiley.
41. Freud, S. 1955. *Group psychology and the analysis of the ego.* Standard Edition, vol. 18. London: Hogarth Press.
42. GAP Report. 1967. Education for community psychiatry. *Group for the Advancement of Psychiatry,* vol. 6, no. 64.
43. ———. 1968. Dimensions of community psychiatry. *Group for the Advancement of Psychiatry,* vol. 6, no. 69.
44. Gaskill, H. S., et al. 1968. Observations on psychiatric residency training in community psychiatry. *Archives of General Psychiatry,* vol. 18 (January).
45. Glasscote, R., et al. 1964. The community mental health center: an analysis of existing centers. Joint Information Service, American Psychiatric Association.
46. ———. 1969. The community mental health center: an interim appraisal. Joint Information Service, American Psychiatric Association.
47. ———. 1969. Partial hospitalization for the mentally ill: a study of programs and problems. Joint Information Service of the American Psychiatric Association and the National Association for Mental Health.
48. Goldston, S. 1964. Training in community psychiatry: a survey report of the medical school departments of psychiatry. *American Journal of Psychiatry,* vol. 120 (February).
49. ———, ed. 1965. Concepts of community psychiatry: a framework for training. Washington, D.C.: U.S. Department of Health, Education and Welfare, Public Health Service Publication No. 1319.
50. Goshen, C. 1959-60. Interdisciplinary trends in mental hygiene research and training. *American Journal of Psychiatry,* vol. 116.
51. Greenblatt, M., Emery, P., and Glueck, B. 1967. Poverty and mental health: implications for training. *Psychiatric Research Reports, American Psychiatric Association,* vol. 21 (January).
52. Hallowitz, E. 1966. The use of indigenous non-professionals in a mental health service. *National Social Welfare Assembly* (September).
53. ———. 1967. The role of a neighborhood service center in a community mental health program. *American Journal of Orthopsychiatry* (April).
54. Hansell, N., Wodarczyk, M., and Visotsky, H. 1968. The mental health expediter. *Archives of General Psychiatry,* vol. 18 (April).
55. Hartman, H. 1958. *Ego psychology and the problem of adaptation.* New York: International Universities Press.
56. Hassler, F. 1965. Psychiatric manpower and community mental

health: a survey of psychiatric residents. *American Journal of Orthopsychiatry,* vol. 35 (July).
57. Hawkinshire, F. 1963. Training needs for offenders working in community treatment programs. In *Experiment in culture expansion.* The National Institute of Mental Health.
58. Hollingshead, A., and Redlich, F. 1958. *Social class and mental illness.* New York: Wiley and Sons.
59. Holt, R. 1959. Personality growth in psychiatric residents. *Archives of General Psychiatry,* vol. 81 (February).
60. Holt, W. 1961. Advances in psychiatric teaching and training programs. *Diseases of the Nervous System,* vol. 22 (February).
61. Holzberg, J., et al. 1964. Chronic patients and a college companion program. *Mental Hospitals,* vol. 15 (March).
62. Hume, P. B. 1964. Community psychiatry, social psychiatry and community mental health work: some interprofessional relationships. *American Journal of Psychiatry,* vol. 121 (October).
63. ——. 1964. Principles and practice of community psychiatry: the role and training of the specialist in community psychiatry. In *Handbook of community psychiatry and community mental health,* ed. Bellak. New York: Grune and Stratton, Inc.
64. Jahoda, M. 1958. *Current concepts of positive mental health.* New York: Basic Books.
65. Joint Commission on Mental Illness and Health. 1961. *Action for mental health.* New York: Basic Books.
66. Jones, M. 1953. *The therapeutic community.* New York: Basic Books.
67. Kantor, D. 1962. Impact of college students on chronic mental patients and on the organization of the mental hospital. In *College student companion program: contribution to the social rehabilitation of the mentally ill.* Connecticut State Department of Mental Health.
68. Kaplan, S. R. 1967. Therapy groups and training groups: similarities and differences. *International Journal of Group Psychotherapy,* vol. 17, no. 4.
69. ——. Psychotherapeutic approaches in working with the disadvantaged. In *Innovations in Psychotherapy,* ed. Goldman G. and Millman, D. Springfield, Ill.: Charles C. Thomas (in press).
70. ——, Boyajian, L., and Meltzer, B. 1969. The role of the nonprofessional worker in disadvantage areas. In *Community mental health practice,* ed. Grunebaum. Boston: Little Brown Co.
71. ——, and Roman, M. 1961. Characteristic responses in adult therapy groups to the introduction of new members: a reflection on group processes. *International Journal of Group Psychotherapy,* vol. 11 (October).
72. ——, and Roman, M. 1963. Phases of development in an adult therapy group. *International Journal of Group Psychotherapy,* vol. 13, no. 1.
73. Kern, H. M., Jr. and Chandler, C. 1960. The cultivation of community mental hygiene leadership ability as part of a psychiatric resident's training. *American Journal of Psychiatry,* vol. 117 (October).

74. ——, et al. 1966. Preparing psychiatric residents for community psychiatry. *Hospital Community Psychiatry,* vol. 17 (December).
75. Knight, J. 1963. Community psychiatry in psychiatric education. *Bulletin of Tulane Medical Faculty,* vol. 22 (May).
76. Komar, M. 1967. A therapeutic community for out-patients. *Mental Hygiene,* vol. 51, no. 3 (July).
77. Kraft, A. 1965. Evaluating the effectiveness of mental health services. *Milbank Memorial Fund Quarterly,* New York.
78. Kraft, A. M., Bennie, P. R., Dickey, B. A. 1968. The chronic patient. In *Community Mental Health,* ed. Williams, R. and Ozarin, L. San Francisco: Jossey-Bass.
79. Lauga, A. et al. 1969. The mental health rehabilitation worker: a new member on the psychiatric team. *Community Mental Health Journal* (February).
80. Lazure, D. 1967. Public Health and the psychiatrist. *Canadian Psychiatric Association Journal* (October).
81. Lemkau, P. 1955. *Mental hygiene in public health.* New York: McGraw-Hill.
82. Lindover, S., Roman, M., and Kaplan, S. R. 1969. The training of the non-professional worker in disadvantaged areas. In *Community mental health practice,* ed. Grunebaum. Boston: Little Brown Co.
83. Linn, L. 1968. The fourth psychiatric revolution. *American Journal of Psychiatry,* vol. 124 (February).
84. Masserman, J. 1963. Psychiatric residency training for public institutional service. *American Journal of Psychiatry,* vol. 119 (May).
85. McGee, R. 1965. The suicide prevention center as a model for community mental health programs. *Community Mental Health Journal,* vol. 1, no. 2.
86. Milbank Memorial Fund. 1962. Proceedings of the 38th Annual Conference: decentralization of psychiatric services and continuity of care. New York.
87. Miller, S., and Riessman, F. 1968. *Social class and social policy.* New York: Basic Books.
88. National Clearing House for Mental Health Information. 1964. Community mental health: individual adjustment or social planning. 9th Inter-American Congress of Psychiatry.
89. ——. 1968. Mental health program reports, no. 2, National Institute of Mental Health.
90. Ozarin, L. 1963. Experiences in teaching community psychiatry to residents. *American Journal of Psychiatry,* vol. 120 (September).
91. Pasamanick, B. 1967. The development of physicians for public mental health. *American Journal of Orthopsychiatry,* vol. 37 (April).
92. Pearl, A., and Riessman, F. 1965. *New Careers for the Poor.* New York: Free Press.
93. Peck, H., Kaplan, S. R., et al. 1965. Small group approaches in a day hospital. *International Journal of Group Psychotherapy,* vol. 15, no. 2.
94. ——, Kaplan, S. R., and Roman, M. 1966. Prevention, treatment and social action: a strategy of intervention in a disadvantaged

urban area. *American Journal of Orthopsychiatry,* vol. 36, no. 1.
95. ——, Roman, M., and Kaplan, S. R. 1967. Community action programs and the comprehensive mental health center. In *Poverty and mental health,* ed. Greenblatt, Emery, and Glueck Jr. Psychiatric Research Reports, American Psychiatric Association.
96. ——, and Kaplan, S. R. 1968. A mental health program for the urban multiservice center. In *Mental health and the community: problems, programs and strategies,* ed. Shore and Mannino. New York: Behavioral Publications.
97. ——, Levin, T., and Roman, M. 1969. The health careers institute: a mental health strategy for an urban community. *American Journal of Psychiatry,* vol. 125, no. 9 (March).
98. Redl, F. 1942. Group emotions and leadership. *Psychiatry,* vol. 5.
99. Reidy, J. 1964. *Zone mental health centers: the Illinois concept.* Springfield, Ill.: Charles C. Thomas.
100. Report of the Conference on Graduate Education. 1963. Training the psychiatrist to meet changing needs. Washington, D.C.: American Psychiatric Association.
101. Rieff, R. 1967. Mental health manpower and institutional change. In *Emergent Approaches to Mental Health Problems,* ed. Cowen, Gardner and Zax. New York: Meredith Publishing Co.
102. Rioch, M. 1967. Pilot projects in training mental health counselors. In *Emergent Approaches to Mental Health Problems,* ed. Cowen, Gardner and Zax. New York: Meredith Publishing Co.
103. Robinson, R., and Roman, M. 1966. New directions for the psychiatric aide. *Nursing Outlook,* vol. 14, no. 2 (February).
104. Rosenbaum, M. 1953. Problems in supervision of residents in psychotherapy. *Archives of Neurology and Psychiatry,* vol. 69.
105. ——, and Zwerling, I. 1964. Impact of social psychiatry. *Archives of General Psychiatry,* vol. 11.
106. Ross, M. 1962. The physician, psychiatry and the public health. *American Journal of Psychiatry,* vol. 119 (December).
107. Saslow, G. 1965. Challenges in undergraduate psychiatric education. *American Journal of Psychiatry,* vol. 21 (January).
108. Scheidlinger, S. 1955. The concept of identification in group psychotherapy. *American Journal of Psychotherapy,* vol. 9.
109. ——. 1964. Identification, the sense of belonging and of identity in small groups. *International Journal of Group Psychotherapy,* vol. 17.
110. ——. 1967. The concept of regression in group psychotherapy. *International Journal of Group Psychotherapy,* vol. 18, no. 1.
111. ——, and Sarcka, A. 1968. A mental health consultation-education program with group service agencies in a disadvantaged community. Presented at the American Orthopsychiatric Association, Chicago.
112. Schwab, J., et al. 1966. Training psychiatric residents in consultation work. *Journal of Medical Education,* vol. 41 (November).
113. Schiff, S., and Kellam, S. 1967. A community-wide mental health program of prevention and early treatment in first grade, *Poverty and Mental Health,* ed. Greenblatt, Emery and Glueck, Jr. Psychiatric Research Reports, APA.

114. Silverman, A. 1965. New horizons in psychiatric education. *American Journal of Psychiatry,* vol. 122 (July).
115. Steiner, J., and Kaplan, S. 1969. Out-patient group work-for-pay activity for chronic schizophrenic patients. *American Journal of Psychotherapy,* vol. 23, no. 3 (July).
116. Ward, C., et al. 1966. Psychiatry residency training: changes over a decade. *American Journal of Psychiatry,* vol. 123 (July).
117. Weinberg, J. 1965. Implications of increasing population for the aged for community mental health service: the psychiatrist's responsibility. *Gerontology,* vol. 5 (June).
118. Whitman, R. 1964. Psychodynamic principles underlying T-Group processes. In *T-Group and Laboratory Method,* ed. Bradford, L. New York: John Wiley.
119. Wilder, J. 1968. A case for a flexible longterm sheltered workshop for psychiatric patients. *American Journal of Psychiatry,* in press, 1968.
120. Williams, R., and Ozarin, L. 1968. *Community mental health.* San Francisco: Jossey-Bass.
121. Wise, H. 1968. The neighborhood medical care demonstration. *Milbank Memorial Fund Quarterly,* vol. 46 (July).
122. Zinberg, N., and Friedman, L. 1967. Problems in working with dynamic groups. *International Journal of Group Psychotherapy,* vol. 17.
123. Zwerling, I., and Wilder, J. 1962. Day hospital treatment for acutely psychotic patients. In *Current Psychiatric Therapies,* ed. Masserman, J. New York: Grune and Stratton.